Collaborative Research in Developmental Therapy: A Model With Studies of Learning Disabled Children

Collaborative Research in Developmental Therapy: A Model With Studies of Learning Disabled Children

Margaret A. Short-DeGraff
Kenneth Ottenbacher
Editors

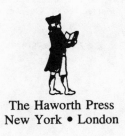

The Haworth Press
New York • London

Collaborative Research in Developmental Therapy: A Model With Studies of Learning Disabled Children is a monographic supplement to the journal *Physical & Occupational Therapy in Pediatrics*, Volume 6, Number 2, Summer 1986. It is not supplied as part of the subscription to the journal, but is available from the publisher at an additional charge.

The Haworth Press, Inc., 28 East 22 Street, New York, NY 10010-6194
EUROSPAN/Haworth, 3 Henrietta Street, London WC2E 8LU England

Library of Congress Cataloging in Publication Data

Collaborative Research in Developmental Therapy.

    "A monographic supplement to the journal Physical & occupational therapy in pediatrics, volume 6, number 2, summer 1986."—T.p. verso.
    Includes bibliographies and index.
    1. Learning disabilities—Diagnosis. 2. Nystagmus. 3. Vestibular apparatus—Diseases. 4. Neuropsychological tests. 5. Vestibular function tests. 6. Sensory-motor integration—Therapeutic use. I. Short-DeGraff, Margaret A. II. Ottenbacher, Kenneth J. [DNLM: 1. Learning Disorders.
W1 PH683P v.6 no. 2 Suppl / WS 110 C641]
RJ496.L4C49   1986   618.92'89   86-11978
ISBN 0-86656-570-1

CONTENTS

Acknowledgements

PART 1

Ottenbacher K, Short MA. Publication Trends in Occupational Therapy.
Reprinted with permission of The American Occupational Therapy Foundation, Inc., from The Occupational Therapy Journal of Research, Vol. 2, No. 2, 1982, pp. 80-88. Copyright © 1982 by The American Occupational Therapy Foundation, Inc.

PART 2

Ottenbacher K. Identifying Vestibular Processing Dysfunction in Learning-Disabled Children.
Reprinted with permission of The American Occupational Therapy Association, Inc., from The American Journal of Occupational Therapy, Vol. 32, No. 4, 1978, pp. 217-221. Copyright © 1978 by The American Occupational Therapy Association, Inc.

Short MA, Watson PJ, Ottenbacher K, Rogers C. Vestibular-Proprioceptive Functions in 4 Year Olds: Normative and Regression Analysis.
Reprinted with permission of The American Occupational Therapy Association, Inc., from The American Journal of Occupational Therapy, Vol. 37, No. 2, February 1983, pp. 102-109. Copyright © 1983 by The American Occupational Therapy Association, Inc.

Clyse SJ, Short MA. The Relationship Between Dynamic Balance and Postrotary Nystagmus in Learning-Disabled Children.
Reprinted with permission of The Haworth Press, Inc., from Physical & Occupational Therapy in Pediatrics, Vol. 3, No. 3, Fall 1983, pp. 25-32. Copyright © 1983 by The Haworth Press, Inc.

PART 3

Ottenbacher K, Watson PJ, Short MA, Biderman MD. Nystagmus and Ocular Fixation Difficulties in Learning-Disabled Children.
Reprinted with permission of The American Occupational Therapy Association, Inc., from The American Journal of Occupational Therapy, Vol. 33, No. 11, November 1979, pp. 717-721. Copyright © 1979 by The American Occupational Therapy Association, Inc.

Ottenbacher K, Watson PJ, Short MA. Association Between Nystagmus Hyporesponsivity and Behavioral Problems in Learning-Disabled Children.
Reprinted with permission of The American Occupational Therapy Association, Inc., from The American Journal of Occupational Therapy, Vol. 33, No. 5, May 1979, pp. 317-322. Copyright © 1979 by The American Occupational Therapy Association, Inc.

PART 4

Watson PJ, Ottenbacher K, Short MA, Kittrell J, Workman EA. Human Figure Drawings of Learning-Disabled Children With Hyporesponsive Postrotary Nystagmus.
Reprinted with permission of The Haworth Press, Inc., from Physical & Occupational Therapy in Pediatrics, Vol. 1, No. 4, Summer 1981, pp. 21-25.

Ottenbacher K. Patterns of Postrotary Nystagmus in Three Learning-Disabled Children.
Reprinted with permission of The American Occupational Therapy Association, Inc., from The American Journal of Occupational Therapy, Vol. 36, No. 10, October 1982, pp. 657-663. Copyright © 1982 by The American Occupational Therapy Association, Inc.

Ottenbacher K, Short MA, and Watson PJ. Nystagmus Duration Changes of Learning-Disabled Children During Sensory Integrative Therapy.
Reprinted with permission of publisher from Perceptual and Motor Skills, Vol. 48, 1979, pp. 1159-1164.

Ottenbacher K, Abbott C, Haley D, Watson PJ. Human Figure Drawing Ability and Vestibular Processing Dysfunction in Learning-Disabled Children.
Reprinted with permission of publisher from Journal of Clinical Psychology, Vol. 40, No. 4, July 1984, pp. 1084-1089.

PART 5

Ottenbacher K, Short MA, Watson PJ. The Effects of a Clinically Applied Program of Vestibular Stimulation on the Neuromotor Performance of Children With Severe Developmental Disability.
Reprinted with permission of The Haworth Press, Inc., from Physical & Occupational Therapy in Pediatrics, Vol. 1, No. 3, Spring 1981, pp. 1-11. Copyright © 1981 by The Haworth Press, Inc.

The authors want to express their gratitude and acknowledge the assistance of:

their colleagues, especially Paul J. Watson, who assumed responsibility for and co-authored many of the articles in this anthology;

the children and parents of the children who participated in the studies reprinted here;

Jane Kittrell, OTR; Mr. J.O. Pierson, Executive Director; and the staff at East

Tennessee Children's Rehabilitation Center, where this research was initiated in 1977; and

the editors, especially Suzann K. Campbell and Irma J. Wilhelm, and the reviewers associated with the journals which originally published the articles included here.

Dr. Short-DeGraff would like to thank Skidmore College's Department of Psychology for assistance with final manuscript preparation. In addition, she would like to acknowledge the support and assistance of Alfred H. DeGraff.

M.A. Short-DeGraff, PhD, OTR/L
Research Fellow, Center for Child Study, Department of Education
Lecturer, Department of Psychology
Skidmore College
Saratoga Springs, New York 12866

K. Ottenbacher, PhD, OTR
Associate Professor
Occupational Therapy Program
School of Allied Health Professions
University of Wisconsin-Madison
Madison, Wisconsin 53706

Collaborative Research in Developmental Therapy: A Model With Studies of Learning Disabled Children

INTRODUCTION

This collection of articles was assembled for many purposes and for many audiences. Interest in clinical research has recently exploded in the allied health fields, and new journals, innovative studies and interdisciplinary collaborations are providing exciting new directions in assessment and treatment. Yet this proliferation of research makes it difficult both for the clinical therapist who lacks either the skills or background to read, understand or conduct research and for the researcher attempting to keep current with and to digest such massive amounts of new data. One area that has exhibited such a proliferation is the assessment and treatment of children with learning disabilities.

The identification of learning disabilities is often difficult. The term learning disabilities represents a very broad category of disorders, and the deficits associated with these disorders often vary from emotional disturbances and academic difficulties to abnormal neurobehavioral symptoms. This latter category of symptoms, sometimes referred to as ''soft'' neurological signs, has recently been used to identify a particular type of learning disability which can be characterized by motor incoordination or clumsiness, abnormal muscle tone, impaired standing or dynamic balance, and deficits in other measures of posture, motor and ocular functions.

THE PURPOSE OF THIS ANTHOLOGY

Most of the studies in this anthology examine these clinical measures in learning disabled children. Thus, one purpose of this collection is to share the results obtained from a series of research by investigators who systematically explored particular deficits found in learning disabled children as well as attempting to predict what would happen to these children when they were started in therapy. Another purpose of this anthology is for the studies to be used didactically as a means of practical advice for other therapists interested in understanding and conducting research in clinical settings. Over the course of many years, we have made mistakes and obtained feedback from many different professionals. We wanted to share some of that feedback as well as our continued enthusiasm for research in the field of learning disabilities. Thus, while the collection of articles is important by itself, we have also included a narrative which discusses problems we had with particular studies as well as giving suggestions, practical advice, and important considerations for those of you who will read this anthology and continue exploring these issues in your own clinical research.

We are excited about this anthology because we feel that our line of research has been deliberate and productive. While some professionals concerned about learning disabled children are aware of one or several of our studies, few have access to all of the studies collected here. The advantage of this collection is that the articles, when viewed together, provide illuminating insights regarding a body of clinical research, the relationships between clinical variables, the measurement of specific forms of learning disability, and the potential for predicting responsiveness of these children to therapy.

This anthology may be useful for both teachers and students. It can be used by itself or as an adjunct to other texts for clinical theory, evaluation and assessment, or for research classes. Key topics in this anthology are: clinical assessment, learning disabilities, sensory integration theory, vestibular and proprioceptive functions, and research methods. We feel that these studies, in collection, say more than the sum of their parts; and we encourage readers to look at them collectively. We have tried to design this anthology to be of use to clinicians and to experienced as well as novice researchers. We have included suggestions for future research in several sections as well as additional references for further study of clinical measures of learning disabled children. We have focused on research topics in our narrative because of our conviction that clinicians need to be informed consumers of research published in their professional journals. An informed consumer will obtain a better understanding of the nature, generalizability, and clinical significance of published work. Finally, we want to encourage other therapists and educators to take advantage of the expertise of their colleagues. Conducting and keeping up with research is often best accomplished by dividing responsibilities and sharing the skills and support of colleagues.

THE BENEFITS OF COLLABORATING

Conducting research, such as many of the studies included here, need not be overwhelming or intimidating. Many educators and therapists, in their everyday activities on the job, conduct mini-research projects. Teachers and clinicians who ask themselves, "Is this therapy effective?", "Are my students progressing?", "Will a different modality be more effective than what the client has been doing in the past?", "Should I increase or decrease the duration of therapy?'', are all conducting research. Research is seeking answers to questions and is a natural part of being an effective clinician and educator.

Many teachers and therapists have the opportunities and ideas for developing some very significant and valuable research projects. Most of us, however, do not have *all* of the skills required to: develop the design for a study, collect the data, analyze the data, determine the results, write up the study and get it together to share in an in-service educational program, a conference, or a journal. This points out the value of collaboration. One of the purposes of this anthology is to demonstrate how a series of published research began with some clinical observations and evolved through the collaborative efforts of several individuals who combined their skills and expertise. Another goal of this collection is to illustrate to other clinicians that they, too, can start their own research the way the authors of this anthology did. Thus, we want to share some of the ins and outs, the politics, the ethics, and some of the personal aspects of clinical research. The purpose of doing this is to provide insight, encouragement, and to emphasize some of the interpersonal dynamics behind getting a successful research project together and off the ground.

HOW DID THE COLLABORATION BEGIN?

The primary collaborators on these studies are Ken Ottenbacher, Peggy Short, and Paul Watson. At the time the collaboration started, Ken was a clinical occupational therapist at East Tennessee Children's Rehabilitation Center (ETCRC) in Knoxville, Tennessee. Peggy was starting her clinical pediatric affiliation as an occupational therapy student at ETCRC, and both she and Paul had completed doctoral studies in experimental (physiological) psychology. Both Peggy and Paul were interested in learning more about clinical research, and Ken was interested in expanding his research skills. Ken's first research article[1] had been written and was on the verge of being published. Ken and Jane Kittrell, then Director of Occupational Therapy at ETCRC, had made a number of observations about some of the children receiving occupational therapy services at the center. Ken's and Jane's ideas came from their personal experiences while evaluating, treating and observing the children as well as from previously published research.

Mutual Interests

The collaboration started primarily because all of us were interested in finding out what was happening to the learning disabled children receiving treatment in our clinic. All of us were interested in isolating some of the factors that might be contributing to effective intervention. Research can be fascinating; it is like searching for pieces to a puzzle and trying to fit the pieces together until finally a partial (and often surprising) picture emerges. The three of us shared that enthusiasm and excitement about asking questions in the clinic. We enjoyed reading about, talking about, and writing about our work. Thus, while one of our goals was to enjoy what we were doing, both in the clinic and during our collaboration, another more practical goal was to develop a viable line of research that could be sustained over a long period of time; divided into responsibilities for each of us; and communicated, if necessary, over a distance. In the last sense, we succeeded, as the research projects continued while one or another of us moved to Arkansas, Missouri, Massachusetts, or Wisconsin.

Planning Immediate and Long-Range Projects

Some of the research questions we developed focused on data that were already accumulated in the children's files in the Center. Fortunately, Mr. Jim Pierson, the director of ETCRC, and the parents of the learning disabled children were very cooperative; and we were able to gain access to records. Other research questions we asked were designed to follow children over the course of therapy. Naturally, these studies took much longer to complete. Periodically, especially at the beginning, the three of us would get together, a three-way think-tank, and we would share ideas, solve problems, divide responsibilities, create new studies, lend support, and develop enough grandiose research projects to keep us occupied for the next three generations! One of the hardest things about designing a research study is keeping it small and manageable. A series of research studies investigating a few variables is more informative than one, huge study looking at too many variables. The latter ends up being confusing and saying too many things at once.

It is easy to give advice. One of the purposes of this anthology is to do that. In many cases we give advice because we learned from our mistakes. This is not an anthology of perfect research that should be emulated. Research is a growing process, and the researcher learns through practice. We learned a lot from our mistakes, and we hope that sharing those may prevent some of you from experiencing the same problems. Our research evolved, and so did our skills. We would like to illustrate some of those points by explaining what kinds of research we conducted, what types of errors we made in constructing our studies, and the nature of collaboration that was able to sustain a line of research despite long distances and varying backgrounds.

HOW DOES RESEARCH GET STARTED?

Published studies usually start with a hunch, a clinical observation, a question, insight, or a desire to follow up other published research. The line of research in this collaboration started with some of Ken's questions; however we could trace Ken's questions to discussions with colleagues or to other research, e.g., Ayres[2] and DeQuiros,[3] whose works are discussed in many of the articles. We could also trace Ayres' and DeQuiros' interests back to other research, thus it is really impossible to pinpoint where ideas begin. So, to keep this within manageable bounds, we will stay within our collaboration and start with Ken's first study (''Identifying vestibular processing dysfunction in learning-disabled children'').[1]

Both Ken and Jane had made numerous observations and discussed what might be happening to their clients during treatment. Many children were referred to the clinic because of learning problems or perceptual-motor deficits. These children were then administered a battery of tests including: the *Southern California Sensory Integrations Tests* (SCSIT);[4] a clinical assessment of balance, muscle tone, ocular preference and other motor functions; the *Southern California Postrotary Nystagmus Test* (SCPNT);[5] draw-a-person test; and others. If evaluations indicated deficits, children were assigned to therapy groups and participated in hour-long sessions of occupational therapy involving sensory integration procedures two to three times per week. This involved a variety of tactile, vestibular-proprioceptive, and sensorimotor experiences with net hammocks, scooter boards, ramps, and obstacle courses, as well as socialization experiences and some table top activities involving multisensory input, number and color recognition, and eye-hand coordination.

Most of the children responded positively to therapy; they seemed to enjoy attending and participating in therapy. But were they improving? How would they improve? Were their grades better in school? Had their behaviors changed at home or in school? Had their learning disabilities or sensory-motor problems changed? How could these changes be measured? How can improvement be measured in the clinic? These are the kinds of questions that therapists and teachers (and also parents and administrators) ask. They are the kinds of questions to which we wanted answers, and they are the kinds of questions that can lead to lifetimes of research.

Value of Clinical Observation

One of the ways that teachers and therapists measure improvement is through observation; their clinical observational skills become sharp, and they perceive even subtle changes in students' or clients' behaviors. Certainly parents note change (or absence of change) in their children's behaviors and report this to teachers, however, we also must have measurable indices of improvement. In the clinic, Ken was trying to find a discrete (i.e., it wouldn't interrupt therapy or be too time-consuming) and quantifiable measure of progress. The Southern California Sensory Integration Tests include an entire subset of sensory and motor tests, but they were not designed for repeated use to gauge progress; so alternative measures needed to be determined. One of these tests was the SCPNT. This is a quickly and easily administered, as well as standardized, test of an individual's ocular movement following rotation on a device similar to a child's sit-and-spin toy. Norms were available for the ages of the children we were seeing in the clinic, and the actual administration of the SCPNT was consistent with other vestibular activities the children were performing as a part of their therapy. Thus, the children and the therapist were not pulled from therapy for testing. Testing did not interfere with therapy, and it was an everyday part of the therapists' and clients' activities.

Many of the learning disabled children in the clinic exhibited very short or no noticeable duration of nystagmus during their intake evaluations. Upon closer observation, many of these same children shared other similar traits: they were clumsy; they often acted out, were boisterous or difficult to calm; they had poor balance and could not maintain anti-gravity postures (i.e., they had difficulty holding their heads, shoulders, arms, and legs up) on the scooter boards; and they *seemed*, as a group, particularly responsive to treatment based on sensory integrative principles. These clinical observations formed the basis for most of the research in this anthology.

Corroboration With Theory

As a research group, we were interested in seeing if these informal observations could be confirmed through systematic examination. Existing research already corroborated some of these observations, *in theory*; we wanted to see if the observations held up experimentally. Thus, this line of research had dual origins. First, it developed from perceptive clinical observations, "hunches" about what was happening to a particular group of clients. Second, the validity of the observations was corroborated by the research and observations of other therapists. This was important because not only could the research address behaviors observed directly in the clinic but also because the line of research already had a tie to previously published work. This would enable us to search existing studies for theoretical bases as well as derive even more predictions by combining our "hunches" with the published observations of other therapists. An exciting aspect about clinical research is that it often addresses not only particular theories but also has important practical applications.

REFERENCES

1. Ottenbacher K: Identifying vestibular processing dysfunction in learning-disabled children. *Am J Occup Ther* 32: 217-228, 1978.

2. Ayres AJ:* *Sensory Integration and Learning Disorders.* Los Angeles, Western Psychological Services, 1972.

3. DeQuiros JB: Diagnosis of vestibular disorders in the learning disabled. *J Learn Disabil* 9: 50-58, 1976.

4. Ayres AJ:* *Southern California Sensory Integration Tests.* Los Angeles, Western Psychological Services, 1972.

5. Ayres AJ: *Southern California Postrotary Nystagmus Test.* Los Angeles, Western Psychological Services, 1975.

---

*Some references have since been updated; however, to keep within the time frame discussed in this text, the older references are used.

PART 1: CLINICAL RESEARCH

TYPES AND TRENDS IN CLINICAL RESEARCH

The first article in this anthology, "Publication Trends in Occupational Therapy" (Reprint 1), has been included for two reasons. First, it contains examples of different categories of research including descriptive, correlational, experimental, quasi-experimental, and practical. These are important to understand when reading or conducting research because they affect the scope and implications of every study. Second, this article is included because it illustrates, in one field, a shift in emphasis in these different categories of research in the past 10 years. Similar shifts can be found in other fields such as nursing, special education, and physical therapy. In all of these fields, growing numbers of books, journal articles, conference reports, and special interest sections are oriented toward encouraging and giving advice for expanding the knowledge base and support for clinical research.

WHAT IS RESEARCH?

Research is a systematic way of finding answers to questions. Those questions can be very complicated or quite simple. Research itself can be very complicated, but it does not have to be. In fact, some of the most sophisticated research uses a very straightforward, logical approach in a simple design. Investigators have different reasons for conducting research, and different systems can be used to answer research questions. Certainly experimental methods exercise the most control, but sometimes rigorous control is not possible in clinic and school environments. Much of research involves hypothesis testing. A hypothesis is a statement of a relationship, and it is a way of asking a question. A hypothesis states a relationship between variables. Variables are events or things that can vary—such as hair color, test grades, precipitation, height, weight, perceptual-motor abilities, balance, or grip.

Informally, therapists conduct their own hypothesis testing as they manipulate different forms of treatment or different modalities (or duration, frequency, intensity of therapy) to meet the needs of different clients. Treatment is often varied for clients, as the therapist "hypothesizes'' that one form of stimulation will be more effective than another. What the clinical researcher does is to carry that process one or two steps farther, by *systematically* investigating those clinical hypotheses.

REASONS FOR RESEARCH

The two primary reasons for conducting research are normative (to describe normal performance) and systematic (to verify a theory). Systematic research tests hypotheses, normative research provides descriptions, and both of these are important goals. Included in this collection are examples of and references for both types of research.

STRATEGIES FOR READING AND KEEPING CURRENT WITH RESEARCH

Even with the different kinds of research, articles published in professional journals have basic similarities. Most articles include an abstract or a summary, a main body, and references. The abstract is a brief précis of the article and is usually included at the beginning of the manuscript, whereas a summary is often found at the end. Some articles include both an abstract and a summary.

Keeping up with the recent proliferation of clinical research is difficult, but interested readers should not become overwhelmed and give up. One of the best strategies for keeping current (but not overloaded) is to periodically scan the professional journals that carry information relevant to your field. Scanning involves reading the table of contents and then reading the abstracts or summaries of articles whose titles appear relevant. If you are then interested in further analyzing, but are unfamiliar with reading research, there are some quick ways to review an article. Most studies have sub-headings, and looking at those often gives a key to the type as well as the direction of the study. A descriptive study, such as a historical report or literature review, includes sub-headings outlining the content of the article; whereas most studies with experimental designs include the following subsections: introduction, procedure or method, results, and discussion.

Scanning a descriptive study involves reading the title, abstract, summary and sub-headings to get a general overview of the article. Scanning an experimental study involves reading the title, abstract, the introduction (which gives the rationale for the study), and the conclusion or discussion (which summarizes and gives the implications of the study's findings). Many readers are intimidated by or are confused by the methodology and results sections of studies, and they get hung up on the meaning of the study because they do not understand the statistics. While the procedure and methods sections are, in many respects, the most important elements of a study, they can be overlooked when scanning for general content. If, however, the study is important to your work, then you need to study it in more depth.

Studying a research article requires several skills, the most important of which is healthy skepticism. Most students feel that if something is in print, then it must be "THE TRUTH". This is not the case with research. Many studies are written to support only one point of view, and systematic research is conducted to test a theory. Theories are ways of organizing information, and research is designed to either support or change that organization. Only one or many viewpoint(s) may be expressed in descriptive articles, and every experimental study contains a margin of error. Thus, studying research requires the recognition that one study, by itself, is inconclusive and can only be evaluated within a context of related research. Reading skeptically involves: studying the writer's theoretical orientation (in the introduction, conclusion, and types of references); analyzing the procedure, asking: Does it make sense? Is there enough information so that I could do the study again, myself?; analyzing the methods and results sections by checking statistics or research design books or discussing the data with colleagues; examining the conclusion section, by looking at whether the author overgeneralizes, or reports the limitations as well as the implications of the study. Last, the references need to be studied. Do they reflect a wide or biased scope? Do the references reflect a variety of authors and journals, including current studies, and are the references accessible, i.e., from other published sources?

For those of you who want to study articles, it may be valuable to request a reprint to put in a reference file. A file is important because it is so easy to forget the location of important articles. Rather than tearing articles out of your journals, you can often obtain a copy of the study by sending a reprint request to the author. Include on a post card the title, journal, and date of the desired article. The author's address is often listed in a footnote on the first or last page of the article. If reprints are not available and you do not want to keep files on separate articles, there is another efficient way to keep track of studies. Each time you read a study that is important, make out an index card with the authors' names, the title, location and date of publication, and a brief statement of the contents. That card can be inserted into an index or computer file under specific topics such as: balance, infant assessments, perceptual-motor tests, sensory integration theory. Then, when you want to refer to certain studies, you can easily determine their location. Your journals remain intact, and you avoid using a large amount of space for filing separate copies of articles. In addition, such index or computer files are convenient for preparing bibliographies for in-service programs or research studies, they are easily purged and alphabetized, and are convenient to store, handle, and to share with colleagues and students.

The following article can be examined for its component parts: title; abstract on the first page; authors' affiliations and addresses in a footnote; introduction; procedure, including different types of research; results; discussion; and references. Many journals also include on the first page of every study, three or four brief descriptors, often termed "key words". In the following study, the key words, "research categories" and "allied health research" give the reader some idea of the emphasis and scope of the study under examination.

Publication Trends
in Occupational Therapy

Kenneth Ottenbacher
Margaret A. Short

ABSTRACT. Articles appearing in the *American Journal of Occupational Therapy* over the past decade were reviewed and categorized according to the nature of the article. Seven categories were identified: descriptive, survey, case and field study, correlational, quasi-experimental, true experimental, and practical. Data analysis revealed that there has been a significant change in the type of articles published before and after 1978. This change appears to be confined to certain categories. Specifically, there has been an increase in articles of a quasi-experimental nature and a decrease in articles of a purely descriptive type. The implications of increased research publications in the occupational therapy literature are discussed.

As the 1980s progress and the allied health fields continue to expand, practitioners and consumers are becoming less content with knowing merely the "how to" of treatment and are becoming increasingly concerned with exploring the "why" of treatment. The field of occupational therapy is developing a wide-based research commitment as a result of the profession's desire to validate, through empirical investigation, the therapeutic effectiveness of its practice (The Foundation, 1979; O'Shea, 1974; West, 1976; Yerxa & Gilfoyle, 1976). At present, however, there does not exist a unified body of evidence supporting many of the practices employed by occupational therapists.

Evidence related to the practice of applied fields is derived from research, and this evidence is accumulated by applying theoretical assumptions to concrete, practical situations and then objectively observing and recording the findings. From the accumulated findings, a body of knowledge is gradually developed and verified for its relevance and practical application. Since the field of occupational therapy lacks a wide body of research validating its therapeutic practices, it sometimes fills this void by "borrowing" research from other disciplines, such as medicine and psychology, and then adapting those procedures to an occupational therapy frame of reference. Although it is sometimes advantageous for fields to use the research data and procedures from related disciplines, it is also necessary for individual fields to develop their own data bases. This is particularly important for occupational therapy, which although progressing, has reportedly been lagging in its research development (The Foundation, 1979).

In addition, the pressure on therapists to improve or maintain the performance of handicapped individuals often predisposes them to employ techniques and procedures that are controversial or that have been inadequately examined. As a result, therapy sometimes becomes treatment based on theory rather than treatment based on researched techiques that rigorously verify its application to varying client populations.

It is essential, therefore, that the field of occupational therapy become self-sufficient in generating its own frame of reference and areas of practice. In the past decade, this need has become increasingly recognized as evidenced by national commitments to promote research within the profession. Since 1970, articles discussing the importance of research began appearing with increasing frequency in the occupational therapy literature (Conine, 1972; Ethridge & McSweeney, 1970a, 1970b, 1971a, 1971b, 1971c, 1971d; The Foundation, 1979; Greenstein, 1980; Hasselkus & Safrit, 1976; Marks, 1980; O'Shea, 1974; West, 1976, 1981; Yerxa & Gilfoyle, 1976). In 1976, the Special Project Award Program of the American Occupational Therapy Foundation (AOTF) was redirected to a National Seminar on Research, which generated a number of recommendations aimed at facilitating the development of research in occupational therapy and which signalled a growing national commitment to the need for research (West, 1976; Yerxa & Gilfoyle, 1976). Since then, there has been a proliferation of research-related activities within the profession. Research seminars sponsored by the AOTF have been instituted as a regular part of the profession's programs, and AOTF funds have been made available for research projects. A nationwide roster of research consultants has been compiled to assist therapists in planning and implementing research projects, and a number of research institutes are now being conducted across the country to encourage cooperative research efforts between clinical and academic therapists. In addition, the AOTF, as a result of a 15-month feasibility study, has recently approved the publication of *The Occupational Therapy Journal of Research* (West, 1980).

The purpose of this article is to ascertain to what extent this national commitment to research has been expressed in the content of occupational therapy publications. In 1970, Ethridge and McSweeney (1970b) stated, "We have noticed that research articles have appeared with increasing frequency over the last 15 years to the present state in which one fully expects to find at least one research article in every issue of the *AJOT*" (p. 491). Has the amount of research literature increased since then? The purpose of this investigation is to examine the nature of occupational therapy research articles published in the *American Journal of Occupational Therapy* (*AJOT*) over the past decade. *AJOT* was chosen because at that time it occupied a unique position as the primary outlet for articles published by occupational therapists.

PROCEDURE

All issues of the *AJOT* from January 1970 to May 1980 were reviewed to determine the nature of articles published during this period. Articles were categorized according to a format adapted from Isaac and Michael (1971). The categories and their operational definitions are described below:

- *Descriptive* (Des): Articles were labeled as descriptive if they systematically described a situation, theory, or areas of interest. Articles that were historical in nature or that reconstructed past events as related to the profession were categorized as descriptive. Review articles were also placed in this category. Numerical data or statistical analyses were not found in any descriptive articles.
- *Survey* (Sur): Survey articles included all those in which the author used some type of measuring instrument or interview technique to gather information that was observational or attitudinal in nature. No attempt was made to control or manipulate variables of interest.
- *Case/Field Studies* (C&F): Case/field study articles included those that intensively studied the background, current status, or therapeutic interactions of an individual or small group of individuals over a period of time. These studies generally employed some type of time series design.
- *Correlational* (Corr): Correlational articles investigated the extent to which variations in one factor or variable corresponded with variations in another factor or variable based on the use of correlational statistics.
- *Quasi-Experimental* (Quasi): Quasi-experimental articles approximated "true" research within the limitations of the setting and research design. Dependent and independent variables were generally clearly identified, and an attempt was made to control and manipulate the variables involved. A statistical analysis of the results was presented.
- *True Experimental* (True): True experimental articles investigated possible cause and effect relationships between independent and dependent variables. Treatment conditions were compared with non-treatment control groups, and random assignment of subjects to groups was clearly specified.
- *Practical* (Prac): Practical articles dealt with new developments or modifications of adaptive devices, splinting techniques, or other rehabilitative equipment. These articles were directly applicable to the clinic environment and did not fit into any of the above categories.

A number of articles or features in the journal were not included in the analysis. Among these were Nationally Speaking, Eleanor Clarke Slagle lectures, editorials, The Student Speaks, reports from association departments or task forces, and minutes of meetings.

A total of 694 *AJOT* articles from January 1970 through May 1980 were reviewed. All articles were reviewed by one rater. A second rater reviewed articles for the years 1973 and 1978. A 94% agreement was obtained between the two ratings.

RESULTS

Since so few true experimental studies were encountered and because they were not numerous enough to comprise a separate percentage category, true experimental figures were combined with the quasi-experimental category. Table 1 presents the results of the article tabulations in percentages according to category for the 10 1/2-year period under study. The percentages for 1980 are included, although they are based on tabulations made for journal articles through May 1980 only.

To further substantiate the descriptive information and to determine if a trend of any statistical significance existed among the categories of articles published in the journal before and after the AOTF made its national commitment to research in 1976 (West, 1976), a chi-square analysis was computed. A 2×6 chi-square was used, with time versus type of article as the cells of the chi-square table. Considering the lag time in publication and the time required to complete a study, it was thought that it would take at least one to one and a half years after the research seminar of 1976 before any changes in the literature might become evident. There-

Table 1

Percent of Articles Published in Each Category by Year

Research Category	1970	1971	1972	1973	1974	1975	1976	1977	1978	1979	1980
Des	57	69	63	38	55	35	63	55	40	39	38
Sur	8	3	11	9	8.5	15	3	8	7	16	13
C&F	4	12	7	16	8.5	9	5	3	10	7	8
Corr	3	3	3	4	4	2	5	5	2	3	4
Quasi	8	5	7	21	11	9	5	7	16	14	29
Prac	20	8	9	12	13	30	19	22	25	21	8
Total number per year	75	75	57	55	71	66	59	73	68	71	24[a]

[a]Includes articles from January through May 1980.

fore, the time factor was divided into two groups, with one group consisting of articles published from 1970 through 1977 and the other group consisting of articles published from 1978 through May 1980. The type of article consisted of the six categories previously described. A X^2 of 16.20 (p < .01, df = 5) was obtained, indicating a significant change in the type of articles published before and after 1978. Visual inspection of the chi-square table revealed that the greatest variation occurred between the two categories of descriptive and quasi-experimental research. Therefore, for further clarification, a second 2 × 2 chi-square was computed using time and only the descriptive versus quasi-experimental categories. This analysis also revealed a significant X^2 of 12.99 (p < .001, df = 1).

A comparison of the percent of quasi-experimental and descriptive articles published each year is illustrated in Figure 1.

DISCUSSION

The results of the chi-square analysis and inspection of Table 1 and Figure 1 reveal that there has been a longitudinal change in the type of articles published in the *AJOT* over the past 10 1/2 years. This change, however, has been confined to certain categories of articles. Specifically, there has been an increase in articles labeled quasi-experimental. These articles, which include the identification of independent and dependent variables and an attempt to manipulate and control variables within the limits of the design and treatment setting, can be seen (in Figure 1) as increasing dramatically from 1978 to the present. It is of interest that an unusually large number of quasi-experimental articles were published in 1973. This may partially be explained by the fact that in 1973 a series of articles appeared in *AJOT* under the heading of "Research in Sensory Integration." This series was the result of a research training workshop (Gilfoyle, 1973) held in 1971-72 and funded by a Maternal and Child Health Services Grant to the Colorado State University's Occupational Therapy Program. This seminar was not directly sponsored or administered by AOTF or the American Occupational Therapy Association (AOTA) and occurred prior to the association's clear-cut commitment to promote research. It should be noted that the increase in quasi-experimental research is due to multiple factors, and, as West (1981) has pointed out:

Research has been conducted by occupational therapists in both intraprofessional investigations and interprofessional, collaborative studies for many years. It cannot, therefore, be claimed that generation of research in the profession began with allocation of funds for research grants by the Association's Representative Assembly in

May 1978. Such a cause-and-effect relationship is suggested only with reference to the impetus that action gave to additional research efforts and involvement by occupational therapists. (p. 7)

While articles of a quasi-experimental type have been increasing, articles of a descriptive nature have correspondingly been declining over the past 10 1/2 years. Other categories, such as correlational or case and field studies, have remained relatively stable. Articles of a true experimental nature were so infrequent that they could not compose a separate category and were included in the quasi-experimental category. It is not unusual that true experimental studies are scarce in a field such as occupational therapy because of the ethical limitations of withholding treatment in order to establish control groups and because of the imposed limitations on random selection of subjects from a clinical setting (Payton, 1980).

As West (1976) and Conine (1972) have pointed out, a profession's base depends on three elements. These are service, training or education, and research. It is encouraging that the field of occupational therapy is ex-

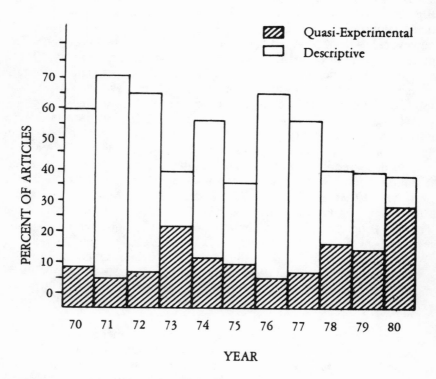

Figure 1   Comparison of Quasi-Experimental and Descriptive Articles Published Over a Ten and a Half Year Period

panding its research base and that this expansion is using more experimental procedures, as illustrated in this study's presentation of the increase of the quasi-experimental category of research. Research, itself, cannot provide final answers to many therapy-related questions, but it can provide definition, support, substantiation, and direction for the implementation of therapies and modalities. It has been illustrated that in an applied field, research can effectively coalesce within a clinic setting to facilitate not only the research base but also the service elements of a profession (Carroll, Miller, Ross & Simpson, 1980). The profession of occupational therapy stands to benefit from the development of its research base in many ways, such as the improvement in the documentation of treatment outcomes, the validation of therapeutic effectiveness for third party payers, and the enhancement of professional and academic identity. In the final analysis, the real beneficiaries of quality research will not be individual therapists, or even the profession itself, but the clients and consumers of occupational therapy practice.

REFERENCES

Carroll, R., Miller, A., Ross, B., & Simpson, G. Research as an impetus to improved treatment. *Archives of General Psychiatry*, 1980, *37*, 377-380.

Conine, T. Dilemmas of research in occupational therapy. *American Journal of Occupational Therapy*, 1972, *26*, 81-84.

Ethridge, D., & McSweeney, M. Research in occupational therapy, Part I: Introduction. *American Journal of Occupational Therapy*, 1970a, *24*, 490-494.

Ethridge D., & McSweeney, M. Research in occupational therapy, Part II: The hypothesis. *American Journal of Occupational Therapy*, 1970b, *24*, 551-555.

Ethridge, D., & McSweeney, M. Research in occupational therapy, Part III: Research design. *American Journal of Occupational Therapy*, 1971a, *25*, 24-28.

Ethridge, D., & McSweeney, M. Research in occupational therapy, Part IV: Data collection and analysis. *American Journal of Occupational Therapy*, 1971b, *25*, 90-97.

Ethridge, D., & McSweeney, M. Research in occupational therapy, Part V: Data interpretation, results and discussion. *American Journal of Occupational Therapy*, 1971c, *25*, 149-154.

Ethridge, D., & McSweeney, M. Research in occupational therapy, Part VI: Research writing. *American Journal of Occupational Therapy*, 1971d, *25*, 210-214.

The Foundation. Research in occupational therapy, it's everybody's responsibility. *American Journal of Occupational Therapy*, 1979, *33*, 666-667.

Gilfoyle, E. Research in sensory integrative development: An introduction. *American Journal of Occupational Therapy*, 1973, *27*, 189-190.

Greenstein, L. Teaching research: An introduction to statistical concepts and research terminology. *American Journal of Occupational Therapy*, 1980, *34*, 320-327.

Hasselkus, B., & Safrit, M. Measurement in occupational therapy. *American Journal of Occupational Therapy*, 1976, *30*, 429-436.

Isaac, S., & Michael, W. *Handbook in research and evaluation.* San Diego, Calif.: EDITS Publications, 1971.

Marks, R. Choosing the appropriate design and analysis of a research project. *Occupational Therapy in Mental Health*, 1980, *1*, 69-76.

O'Shea, B. Why research? *Canadian Journal of Occupational Therapy*, 1974, Autumn, 78-81.

Payton, O. D. *Research: The validation of clinical practice.* Philadelphia: F. A. Davis, 1980.

West, W. Nationally speaking: Research seminar. *American Journal of Occupational Therapy*, 1976, *30*, 477-478.

West, W. Foundation to publish O. T. journal of research. *Occupational Therapy Newspaper*, December 1980, *34*, p. 1.

West, W. Commentary: A journal of research in occupational therapy: The response, the responsibility. *Occupational Therapy Journal of Research*, 1981, *1*, 7-12.

Yerxa, E., & Gilfoyle, E. The Foundation: Research seminar. *American Journal of Occupational Therapy*, 1976, *30*, 509-514.

PART 2:
INITIAL INVESTIGATIONS:
RELATIONS AMONG VARIABLES

To start research with a rigorous experimental method in a fairly new field is difficult. Relationships between variables cannot be hypothesized until the specific variables are recognized. Frequently, initial research projects involve discovering variables on which to focus. In the following three studies, this was done. The first study "Identifying Vestibular Processing Dysfunction in Learning-Disabled Children" (Reprint 2) was Ken's attempt to see what clinical variables related to one another. In the Introduction to this anthology, we discussed the clinical observations regarding children with low (or zero) nystagmus who seemed to show other clinical signs such as poor balance and anti-gravity postures. This first study was an attempt to explore those observations systematically, to determine which variables were related and which variables were good predictors of nystagmus. In a sense, the first study does test a hypothesis. Ken had hypothesized that, in learning disabled children, the clinical measures of nystagmus, muscle tone, balance, and other postures would show a positive relationship to one another. As we pointed out in the Introduction, this study had its origins not only in clinical observations but also in other published research. The introduction of this specific study indicates that work by Ayres[1] and DeQuiros[2] provided an important research foundation.

CORRELATIONAL STUDIES

The three studies collected in this section certainly have experimental methodologies, i.e., they are systematic; however, experimental designs were not used. The studies can be considered exploratory, attempting to discover relations among variables. All three studies in this section have correlational designs (or use correlational statistics) for examining multiple relations among variables. In all of the studies multiple regression was used. Although this is a complicated statistical procedure, it is merely a method for looking at many variables, all at once, and seeing how much they relate to one another, i.e., co-vary. Usually, the experimenter has one variable that is of interest, and that variable is held stable while the others are compared to it. This stable variable is called a criterion variable and, in most of these studies, the criterion variable is the duration of postrotary nystagmus, as measured by standardized procedures on the SCPNT.[3]

Correlational designs have drawbacks. They are informative for preliminary analyses, but experimental designs offer more control and subsequently more understanding about the variables under investigation. One of the drawbacks to correlational studies is the limited conclusions that can be drawn. A correlation shows relation but not causation. When variables are found to co-vary, we know that they both change in relation to one another, but what causes this change is not known. The cause may be some totally extraneous factor(s). For example, the amount of dirt and road salt on your car and the amount of antihistamines you need for a cold may correlate—not because one causes the other but because both may be connected to cold, snowy weather.

Taken together, two of the following three articles show that nystagmus, muscle tone, and balance are correlated in a population of learning disabled children. From this we may safely conclude that, in this population, a proportion of learning disabled children with low durations of nystagmus also evidence hypotonia and poor balance, but this does not say that low nystagmus *causes* low muscle tone or inadequate balance. Although the conclusions that can be drawn from correlational studies are limited, other research that lends support to these conclusions should not be disregarded.

Clinical theorists speculate that perhaps all of these variables (low nystagmus, hypotonia and poor balance) result from an immature or deficient vestibular system.[1] Theory, however, is a way of organizing information but it may or may not be accurate. That is the value of research—to test and either support or amend theory. The results from the studies in this section certainly lend support to the theory that these specific clinical variables are related and *may* reflect an immature vestibular apparatus or an inability to adequately process vestibular-related information; but the results from these studies can be interpreted in other ways as well. For example, the variables may reflect, not a deficient vestibular apparatus, but instead, level of arousal,[4] motivation, or some other extraneous variable. Thus, the correlational analyses made here are, in a sense, preliminary. They can be very important and suggest numerous directions for future study, but they do not pinpoint causes. Experimental designs, on the other hand, tend to offer more solid tests of theory.

The second study in this section "Vestibular-proprioceptive Functions in 4 Year Olds: Normative and Regression Analyses" (Reprint 3), is an extension of Ottenbacher's 1978 work with an additional approach. The children in the study by Short and associates were not learning disabled clients in a clinic but instead consisted of four-year-old Head Start participants. Since little focus has been directed at this age group, we decided that descriptive data would be useful for other therapists working with similar populations. Thus, two purposes were assigned to this project: to study the relations among clinical variables as Ken had previously done and to provide normative data regarding clinical assessment of a preschool population.

COLLECTING DATA AS A PART OF DAILY ROUTINE

Both studies mentioned so far were conducted as a part of the therapists' regular daily activities. Ken's study was based on data accumulated as the clients entered the clinic, and the data in the study by Short and associates were accumulated as a Head Start requirement to assess all children's abilities at the beginning of school.

MODELING A PREVIOUS STUDY

The third study "The Relationship Between Dynamic Balance and Postrotary Nystagmus in Learning Disabled Children" (Reprint 4) by Clyse and Short, illustrates how one study can serve as a springboard for another research project. As a graduate student at Boston University, Sally Clyse became interested in the research that is now accumulated in this anthology. The results of Ken's 1978 study had indicated that certain variables were related to one another. All of these variables are, in theory, vestibular-related. Sally wondered whether other variables that would offer greater challenge to the vestibular system would be even more strongly related. She decided to use almost the same procedure that Ken had used in the 1978 study except that she included an investigation of dynamic balance. While this is not an exact replication, parts of her study replicated previous work.

Basing research on previous studies has many advantages. You can learn from the previous investigators' errors, you can use the exact same procedure, and you can use many of the same references. Many new researchers think that they need to carve out entirely new areas of investigation, but this is not true. The most conclusive and definitive areas of research are ones where many investigators, from varying disciplines and geographical regions, have examined similar variables, over and over, using similar designs and changing only a few variables or the type of subject population each time. Conclusions from any one study should be considered tentative. The strength of research lies in repetition and replication.

DRAWING CONCLUSIONS

The results from the Clyse and Short study were satisfying to us because in general they confirmed Ken's finding regarding the relationships of certain clinical variables to nystagmus duration. Additional findings indicated that a measure of dynamic balance, easily administered in the clinic, was a stronger predictor of nystagmus than was standing balance and that balance measures with the eyes closed seemed to be stronger predictors of nystagmus than were balance measures with the eyes open. We stated in the previous paragraph, however, that conclusions from one study should be tentative. For example, Short and associates caution that different clinical assessments have varying utility with different age populations. Hyperextended prone extension is very difficult for four-year-old children, whereas it may be a good discriminator for teen-aged learning disabled children. While Clyse and Short found relationships between variables similar to what Ottenbacher had reported, Short and associates did not find those relationships within a population of Head Start children. Certain variables may be good discriminators for some learning disabled populations but not for others.

A good *body* of research looks at similar variables, in many different circumstances, and with many different populations. An example of this is the normative data that are accumulating in regard to postrotary nystagmus (prn). At present, a number of studies give insight and also suggest numerous future research projects examining factors influencing prn. Some of those factors may be sex, race, geographical location, arousal, age, or kind of disability. The work by Ayres;[3] Crowe, Deitz and Siegner;[4] Deitz and Crowe;[5] Deitz, Siegner and Crowe;[6] Kimball;[7] Montgomery and Capps;[8] Montgomery and Rodel;[9] Morrison and Sublett;[10] Punwar;[11] Utley, Pettit and Robertson;[12] Zee-Chen and Hardman;[13] and others gives us numerous suggestions for further systematic and normative research studies. Additionally, explorations of clinical variables such as the work by Bundy and Fisher,[14] Dunn,[15] Dutton,[16] Gregory-Flock and Yerxa,[17] Harris,[18] Montgomery,[19] and others will help not only in clarifying relationships among variables but also enhance subsequent assessments of balance and other vestibular-related factors.

RESEARCH IDEAS

In regard to future research, the three studies included here pose numerous possibilities for both systematic and normative approaches. Examples of research questions that can be asked are: Are any other variables *better* predictors of low nystagmus? In what populations? What other characteristics are found in children with low nystagmus? What is the relationship between performance on static and dynamic balance assessments in learning disabled children? Is there an age at which dynamic balance is too difficult for children and is not useful as a clinical measure? What happens to each of the clinical variables, isolated *and* in combination, when different kinds (or ages) of learning disabled populations are exposed to therapy? What therapy is most effective? Is therapy most effective at a certain age? Do certain, specific populations respond more to specific interventions? What is the best method, duration, and order for administering that intervention? A few of these questions are addressed in the following section.

REFERENCES

1. Ayres AJ: *Sensory Integration and Learning Disorders.* Los Angeles, Western Psychological Services, 1972.
2. DeQuiros JB: Diagnosis of vestibular disorders in the learning disabled. *J Learn Disabil* 9:50-58, 1976.
3. Ayres AJ: *Southern California Postrotary Nystagmus Test: Manual.* Los Angeles, Western Psychological Services, 1975.
4. Crowe TK, Deitz JC, Siegner CB: Postrotary nystagmus response of normal four-year-old children. *Phys Occup Ther Pediatr* 4(2):19-28, 1984.
5. Deitz J, Crowe TK: Developmental status of children exhibiting postrotary nystagmus durations of zero seconds. *Phys Occup Ther Pediatr* 5(2/3):69-80, 1985.
6. Deitz J, Siegner C, Crowe T: The Southern California Postrotary Nystagmus Test: Test-retest reliability for preschool children. *Occup Ther J Res* 1:165-177, 1981.
7. Kimball JG: Normative comparison of the Southern California Postrotary Nystagmus Test: Los Angeles vs. Syracuse data. *Am J Occup Ther* 35:21-25, 1981.
8. Montgomery PD, Capps MJ: Effect of arousal on the nystagmus response of normal children. *Phys Occup Ther Pediatr* 1(2):17-29, 1980.
9. Montgomery PC, Rodel DM: Effect of state on nystagmus duration on the Southern California Postrotary Nystagmus Test. *Am J Occup Ther* 36:177-182, 1982.
10. Morrison D, Sublett J: Reliability of the Southern California Postrotary Nystagmus Test with learning-disabled children. *Am J Occup Ther* 37:694-698, 1983.
11. Punwar A: Expanded normative data: Southern California Postrotary Nystagmus Test. *Am J Occup Ther* 36:183-187, 1982.
12. Utley E, Pettit E, Robertson D: Southern California Postrotary Nystagmus Test: Adult normative data. *Occup Ther Ment Health* 3:29-34, 1983.
13. Zee-Chen EL, Hardman ML: Postrotary nystagmus response in children with Down's Syndrome. *Am J Occup Ther* 37:260-265, 1983.
14. Bundy AC, Fisher AG: The relationship of prone extension to other vestibular functions. *Am J Occup Ther* 35:782-787, 1981.
15. Dunn W: *A Guide to Testing Clinical Observations in Kindergartners.* Rockville MD: American Occupational Therapy Association, 1981.
16. Dutton RE: Reliability and clinical significance of the Southern California Postrotary Nystagmus Test. *Phys Occup Ther Pediatr* 5(2/3):57-64, 1985.
17. Gregory-Flock JL, Yerxa EJ: Standardization of the prone extension postural test on children ages 4 through 8. *Am J Occup Ther* 38:187-194, 1984.
18. Harris NP: Duration and quality of the prone extension position in four-, six-, and eight-year-old normal children. *Am J Occup Ther* 35:26-30, 1981.
19. Montgomery P: Assessment of vestibular function in children. *Phys Occup Ther Pediatr* 5(2/3):33-49, 1985.

Identifying Vestibular Processing Dysfunction in Learning-Disabled Children

Kenneth Ottenbacher

ABSTRACT. The purpose of this investigation was to identify neurobehavioral functions of the vestibulo-proprioceptive system that would aid the clinician in evaluating vestibular processing dysfunction in learning-disabled children. Nine variables identified as related to vestibulo-proprioceptive function were subjected to multiple regression analysis. Data analysis revealed that four variables shared significant variance with Southern California Postrotary Nystagmus Test scores. It is suggested that these variables can provide additional information in evaluating vestibular processing dysfunction in learning-disabled children.

The Brain constructs its systems to enclose
The study paradox of thought and sense;
Momentously its tissued meaning grows
To solve and integrate experience
                                    S. Kunitz

REVIEW OF THE LITERATURE

Considerable controversy in the literature continues concerning the nature of a neurobehavioral substrate in learning disabilities.[1] Nevertheless, the diagnosis under various rubrics is clinically employed to categorize a group of children of grossly normal intelligence showing one or more behavioral abnormalities. Research to identify a neurobehavioral basis for learning disabilities has progressed rapidly during the past decade. Continued empirical investigation is necessary to further delineate the various aspects of learning disabilities and to identify appropriate therapeutic interventions.

There appears to be a growing realization among various professionals that learning disabilities represent more than one clinical entity.[2-4] In more than 15 years of applied research, Ayres has identified and elucidated various neurobehavioral syndromes evidenced by learning-disabled children.[5-7] Disorders in "postural and bilateral integration" was one of several syndromes identified by Ayres in the late sixties through factor analysis procedures.[8] The syndrome as originally described was partially characterized by poorly integrated postural mechanisms, and included evidence of remnants of primitive postural reflexes, poor equilibrium reactions, and poor ocular control.[5] Muscle hypotonia was often found to accompany the syndrome.[5,8] All of these symptoms are associated with the vestibulo-proprioceptive system. The vestibulo-proprioceptive system may be generally defined as that system which regulates posture, tonus, and equilibrium through integration of afferent and efferent information. The introduction of Ayres' *Southern California Postrotary Nystagmus Test* (SCPNT) has quantitatively identified dysfunction of the vestibular system in some children with learning disabilities.[9] Recently, Ayres reported, "The most important finding centered on the vestibular system. About half of the learning-disabled children tested demonstrated shortened duration nystagmus indicating a considerable frequency of inadequate processing of vestibular input."[10,p iii]

In a number of investigations dating from the early 1960s, DeQuiros has identified a disorder in learning disabled children he terms "vestibulo-proprioceptive disintegration."[11] He has performed neurolabyrinthine studies on a large number of children (1,900) from infancy to adolescence with wide-ranging medical diagnoses. In studies he conducted in the mid-sixties, he found more than 50 percent of the children diagnosed as learning disabled had vestibular hyporeflexia to caloric stimulation. DeQuiros identified two syndromes of "vestibulo-proprioceptive disintegration" based on severity of dysfunction. Among the characteristics of both syndromes are muscle hypotonia and lack of vestibular reaction to caloric stimuli.[11] DeQuiros concluded a summary of his research by stating "vestibular disorders can produce learning disabilities associated with motor skills, the acquisition of language and the development of normal competencies in reading-writing."[12,p55]

In studying the achievement of motor milestones in children with sensorineural hearing loss and vestibular dysfunction, Rabin found that many of the subjects had a history of muscle hypotonia together with delays in motor development.[13] Recent research demonstrated statistically significant therapeutic effects of "vestibular stimulation" on the reflex and motor development of normal and developmentally delayed infants and young children.[14-17]

Occupational therapists evaluate and treat children for sensory integrative dysfunction and related perceptual-motor problems. The identification of those children who could benefit from sensory integrative therapy is of primary concern to therapists. Ayres' research referred to above found that "a highly specific therapeutic program in sensory processing ameliorates the dysfunction identified by hyporeactive nystagmus and promotes efficiency of academic learning.''[10,piv] Thus, sensory integrative therapy was found to have a significant therapeutic effect on those children identified as having disorders in processing vestibular information. Measurement of inadequate processing of vestibular information was dependent upon the results of the SCPNT that measures vestibulo-ocular reflex (nystagmus) to rotatory stimulation.[9] It has long been known that various factors, including visual fixation and arousal level, can dramatically effect postrotatory nystagmus resulting from stimulation of the vestibular system.[18] Research has shown that in some normal subjects the presence of light in the visual field is sufficient to result in a visual fixation that may significantly suppress vestibular nystagmus.[19] The possible variations in vestibular nystagmus due to variables not controlled in the SCPNT,[9] the relative importance of SCPNT scores in the interpretation of the *Southern California Sensory Integration Tests* (SCSIT),[20] and in identifying those children most likely to benefit from sensory integrative therapy[10] provided the impetus for this investigation. The purpose of this study was to further identify the neurobehavioral aspects of vestibular processing that may be related to postrotatory nystagmus. An attempt was made to determine to what degree SCPNT scores would be related to clinical observations and standardized tests commonly employed by occupational therapists in evaluating children identified as learning disabled. It was hypothesized that a significant relationship would exist between SCPNT scores and estimation of muscle tone.

PROCEDURE

This was a retrospective study in the sense that the various measurements used as variables were administered over a 16-month period as a service to the subjects at a children's rehabilitation center. The subjects consisted of 73 males and 19 females between 53 and 120 months of age. These 92 children were subjects with a medical and educational diagnosis of learning disabilities, minimal brain dysfunction, or perceptual-motor disorder screened from a larger sample of 138. All subjects were without overt physical or mental handicaps. IQs were within a normal range as far as could be determined from school and psychological reports.

The subjects were individually administered the SCSIT, the SCPNT, and an informal assessment of postural mechanisms and reflex integration by two therapists experienced in sensory integration theory and practice, one of whom was certified in administration and interpretation of the SCSIT.

The variables used for data analysis included scores from the following standardized tests: SCPNT ($\bar{x}$ 33.17; SD 7.64) and the Standing Balance Eyes Open (SBO) ($\bar{x}$ 43.01); SD 9.15), Standing Balance Eyes Closed

(SBC) ($\bar{x}$ 39.81; SD 11.46) tests of the SCSIT. All means ($\bar{x}$) and standard deviations (SD) of standardized tests are reported as T-scores. Administration of these tests was in accordance with standardized instructions in the respective manuals (9,21). In addition, the following variables were obtained from clinical assessment of postural mechanisms and reflex integration; muscle tone ($\bar{x}$ 2.12; SD .81), prone extension posture ($\bar{x}$ 1.91; SD .80), supine flexion posture ($\bar{x}$ 2.36; SD .54), muscle co-contraction ability ($\bar{x}$ 2.64; SD .56), age ($\bar{x}$ 83 mo; SD 19.12), and sex. The method of evaluating and scoring these variables was adapted from Ayres[8] and appears in the *Appendix*. The particular variables chosen were based on a review of the literature and upon clinical experience identified as being related to vestibulo-proprioceptive functions. Interrater reliability coefficients were computed for 12 subjects on each of the 9 variables excluding sex and age and resulted in *r* variables ranging from .78 to .98.

RESULTS

Examination of the data showed a tendency for those subjects with depressed nystagmus scores (< −1.0) to evidence some degree of hypotonicity, whereas those subjects with normal or above postrotatory nystagmus were more likely to have normal muscle tone. Forty-six percent of the subjects had SCPNT scores of less than − 1.0. Twenty-two percent had muscle tone that was definitely hypotonic.

A *chi*-square for independence was computed between estimation of muscle tone and SCPNT scores with a resultant $X^2 = 30.45$. The null hypothesis that muscle tone and SCPNT scores are independent was rejected at the $p < .001$ level.

Multiple regression equations were generated for specific dependent variables using a program with subsets developed according to Schatzoff and others.[22] SCPNT scores of less than − 1.0 and greater than + 1.0 are interpreted as abnormal, although probably measuring different aspects of neurovestibular dysfunction.[9] This variable was therefore coded as a dummy variable with three categories: scores less than − 1.0, scores between − 1.0 and + 1.0, and scores greater than + 1.0. Sex was also coded as a dummy variable. Dummy variable coding is used to render the information of membership in one group by a series of *g*-1 dichotomies. Since each dummy variable is a dichotomy, it expresses one meaningful aspect of group membership with the dependent variable of the sample. Variable coding was performed according to Cohen.[23]

Generation of the regression equation yields an R^2 that equals the proportion of the variance of the dependent variable accounted for by the independent variables. For example, for the dependent variable *muscle tone*, a multiple regression equation was generated that included the remaining independent variables: prone extension posture, supine flexion posture, muscle co-contraction, SBO, SBC, SCPNT, age, and sex. The R^2 for this particular equation was .6084. Thus, approximately 61 percent of the variance of the dependent variable (muscle tone) was accounted for by the independent variables.

In order to determine which of the independent variables contributed most to the variance shared with the different dependent variables, the regression coefficients from the independent variables were converted to beta weights. A list of the significant beta weights computed from the independent variables for each dependent variable is shown in Table 1. The independent variable that has the largest absolute beta weight contributes the most to the variance shared with the dependent variable, or is the best predictor of that dependent variable. Conversely, a small beta weight indicates that the corresponding independent variable is not contributing to shared variance, or prediction, as much as the other independent variables. For example, for the dependent variable of *muscle tone*, the independent variable of muscle co-contraction has the largest absolute beta weight and thus shared the greatest amount of variance, or was the best predictor of muscle tone. SCPNT, prone extension posture, and age, respectively, were the three next independent variables that shared the largest amounts of variance with, or were the best predictors of, muscle tone.

DISCUSSION AND CONCLUSION

The hypothesis that muscle tone and SCPNT scores would be related was confirmed. This result further corroborates research findings reported in the literature. The second purpose of this investigation was to determine which of the selected variables assumed to measure various aspects of vestibulo-proprioceptive functions would be related to SCPNT scores.

The vestibulo-proprioceptive system has various functional implications in a number of areas associated with learning and postural problems in children identified as learning disabled.[5,12,20] The independent variables of SCPNT and age shared the greatest variance with the dependent variables. In order of greatest shared variance with SCPNT scores the dependent variables were: prone extension posture, SBC, muscle tone, and SBO. All of these variables, except prone extension posture, also shared a significant amount of variance with age. It is interesting to note that SCPNT did not share a significant amount of variance, or prediction, with supine flexion posture. This appears to indicate that, although prone extension posture and supine flexion posture share significant variance with each other, prone extension posture is a more direct indicator of

Table 1

Beta Weights

				Independent Variables					
	MsT	PEP	SFP	CC	SBO	SBC	SCPNT	AGE	SEX
MsT	—	.2580	—	.4064	—	—	.3185	.1408	—
PEP	.2792	—	.4614	—	—	—	.3513	—	—
SFP	—	.4304	—	.1071	—	—	—	.2391	.1198
CC	.5767	—	.1002	—	—	—	—	.1327	—
SBO	—	.3419	—	—	—	.4767	.2444	.1654	—
SBC	.1880	—	—	—	.3875	—	.3200	.2313	—

(Dependent Variables on left axis)

All values reported significant at $p < .01$ ($df/82$).

vestibular processing functions. There is tentative support for this inference in the literature.[20] SCPNT scores shared the greatest variance, or were the best predictors of prone extension posture. Prone extension posture also appeared to be the dependent variable least affected by age. Clinically, this appears to indicate that prone extension posture may be a valuable addition to the assessment of vestibulo-proprioceptive dysfunction in learning-disabled children. It is suggested that all dependent variables identified as sharing significant variance with SCPNT should be routinely included in clinical evaluation of the vestibulo-proprioceptive system.

The data analytical spirit in which this investigation was undertaken provides the researcher with "indications" rather than "conclusions."[24] Although multiple regression is a very flexible data analytical system, the "indications" provided by this study must be viewed as tentative and oversimplified.

APPENDIX

1. *Muscle Tone* (MsT): The degree of muscle tone was evaluated by passively extending the joints of the upper extremities. Scoring was on a 3-point scale, with 1 = definite hypotonicity, 2 = slight hypotonicity, 3 = normal.
2. *Prone Extension Posture* (PEP): The subject was requested to lie prone and maintain a hyperextended posture with legs, arms (flexed), and head held above the supporting surface. Scoring was

on a 3-point scale, with 1 = unable to assume and maintain posture, 2 = assume and maintain posture for 1-19 seconds, 3 = assume and maintain posture for more than 20 seconds.

3. *Supine Flexion Posture* (SFP): The subject was requested to lie supine and maintain a completely flexed posture with legs, arms, and head in flexion and held above the supporting surface. Scoring was on a 3-point scale, with 1 = unable to assume and maintain posture, 2 = assume and maintain posture 1-19 seconds, 3 = assume and maintain posture for more than 20 seconds.

4. *Muscle Co-Contraction* (CC): The subject was requested to maintain body segments in a rigid posture by simultaneous contraction of antagonistic muscle groups while the examiner applied alternating resistance. Scoring was on a 3-point scale, with 1 = definite deficiency, 2 = slight deficiency, 3 = normal.

5. *Sex*: Scored on a 2-point scale, with 1 = male, 2 = female.

REFERENCES

1. Vellutioni F, et al: Has the perceptual deficit hypothesis led us astray. *J Learn Disabil* 10:6, 1977

2. Walzer PH, Wolff P: *Minimal Cerebral Dysfunction in Children,* New York: Grune and Stratton, 1973

3. Wender P: *Minimal Brain Dysfunction in Children*, New York: Wiley-Interscience, 1971

4. Mallinger, B: Background interference procedures and discriminant function analysis in predicting clinically determined categories of learning disability. *J Percept Mot Skills* 44:767-776, 1977

5. Ayres AJ: *Sensory Integration and Learning Disorders*, Los Angeles: Western Psychological Services, 1972

6. Ayres AJ: *The Development of Sensory Integrative Theory and Practice*, Dubuque, IA: Kendall/Hunt Publishing Co., 1974

7. Ayres AJ: Cluster analyses of measures of sensory integration. *Am J Occup Ther* 31:362-366, 1977

8. Ayres AJ: Deficits in sensory integration in educationally handicapped children. *J Learn Disabil* 2:160-168, 1969

9. Ayres AJ: *Southern California Postrotary Nystagmus Test*, Los Angeles: Western Psychological Services, 1975

10. Ayres AJ: *The Effect of Sensory Integrative Therapy on Learning Disabled Children*, Pasadena, CA: Center for Study of Sensory Integrative Dysfunction, 1976

11. DeQuiros JB: Vestibulo-Proprioceptive Integration: Its Influence on Learning and Speech in Children, *Proc 10th Interam Cong & Psychol*, Lima, Peru, 1966, Trillas, Mexico, 1967

12. DeQuiros JB: Diagnosis of vestibular disorders in the learning disabled. *J Learn Disabil* 9:50-58, 1976

13. Rabin I: Hypoactive labyrinths and motor development. *Clinical Pediatr* 13:922-937, 1974

14. Clark D, Kreutzberg J, Chee F: Vestibular stimulation, influence on motor development in infants. *Science* 196:1228-1229, 1977

15. Clark D, Kantner R: Effects of vestibular stimulation on nystagmus response and motor performance in the developmentally delayed infants. *Phys Ther* 56:414-421, 1976

16. Chee F: *Effects of Vestibular Stimulation on Motor Development in Cerebral Palsied Children*, Master's Thesis, Columbus: Ohio State University, 1975

17. Rogos R: *Clinically Applied Vestibular Stimulation and Motor Performance in Children with Cerebral Palsy*, Master's Thesis, Columbus: Ohio State University, 1976

18. Cogan D: *Neurology of the Ocular Muscles*, 2nd Edition. Springfield, IL: Charles C Thomas, 1956

19. Levy D, Proctor L, Holzman P: Visual interference on vestibular response. *Arch Otolaryngal* 103:287-291, 1977

20. Ayres AJ: *Interpreting the Southern California Sensory Integration Tests*, Los Angeles: Western Psychological Services, 1976

21. Ayres AJ: *Southern California Sensory Integration Tests*, Los Angeles: Western Psychological Services, 1972

22. Schatzoff G, Feinberg E, Tsao E: Efficient calculation of all possible regressions. *Technometrics* 10:4, 769-779, 1968

23. Cohen J, Cohen P: *Applied Multiple Regression/Correlation Analysis for the Behavioral Sciences*, New York: John Wiley and Sons, 1975

24. Tuckey J: The future of data analysis. *Ann Math Stat* 33:1-67, 1962

Vestibular-Proprioceptive Functions in 4 Year Olds: Normative and Regression Analyses

Margaret A. Short
P. J. Watson
Kenneth Ottenbacher
Charlotte Rogers

ABSTRACT. Normative data were obtained for 156 pre-school children's performances on measures of muscle tone, muscle co-contraction, standing balance, prone extension posture, flexion supine posture, asymmetrical tonic neck reflex, and postrotary nystagmus. Regression analysis indicated that these combined variables accounted for only 13.5 percent of the variance of post-rotary nystagmus of 145 four year olds. However, if the data are examined only for children exhibiting nystagmus that is lower than 1 standard deviation below the mean, then these variables account for 50 percent of the variance of nystagmus. Prone extension posture, standing balance-eyes closed, and muscle tone account for 37 percent of the variance within this low-nystagmus population. These results are considered in light of the authors' previous studies demonstrating that, in learning disabled children, vestibular-proprioceptive measures can be used clinically to predict which children will respond to sensory integration therapy with changes in postrotary nystagmus. These changes, according to sensory integration theory, reflect positive responses to therapy.

The early identification of handicapping conditions has received considerable recent focus; however, normative data and standardized evaluations for the assessment of children aged 4 years and younger are still lacking. This lack is particularly evident in the assessment of learning disabilities, which encompass conditions such as perceptual handicaps, brain injury, minimal brain dysfunction, dyslexia, and developmental aphasia.[1,2] The deficits associated with these conditions vary from emotional disturbances and academic difficulties to abnormal neurobehavioral symptoms. This latter category, sometimes referred to as "soft" neurological signs, includes motor incoordination or clumsiness, abnormal muscle tone, impaired balance, and other measures of vestibular and proprioceptive functions.[3] These soft signs serve as aids in the identification of subcategories of learning disabilities.[4]

Because the term *learning disabilities* represents a broad category of diverse disorders, its usefulness as a diagnostic criterion has been criticized.[5] Research has been aimed at identifying subcategories, or syndromes of learning disabilities.[6] The Southern California Postrotary Nystagmus Test (SCPNT)[7] is one index that has proved useful for elucidating these subcategories. The SCPNT is a standardized test that measures the duration of ocular movement (nystagmus) following rotation. Using the SCPNT, Ottenbacher[8] demonstrated that, in school-age children diagnosed as exhibiting learning disabilities, minimal brain dysfunction, or perceptual motor disorders, the duration of postrotary nystagmus (PRN) is directly related to other "soft" neurological signs or measures of vestibular and proprioceptive function. Using these "soft" measures of standing balance, muscle tone, and prone extension posture, Ottenbacher, Short, and Watson[9] were able to predict which learning-disabled children with low postrotary nystagmus would respond with duration increases following sensory integrative therapy (SIT).

The measure of PRN has thus proven useful (1) for the delineation of specific subgroups of school-age learning-disabled children who will respond to therapy, and (2) in combination with four other measures, for prediction of the low-nystagmus learning-disabled children who will respond with duration increases following SIT. Change in the duration of PRN is an important goal of SIT,[10] which has been found effective in ameliorating the academic deficits of learning-disabled children displaying hyperreactive PRN:[11] however, depressed nystagmus can be caused, not only by vestibular processing deficits,[10] but also by visual fixation, by reductions in arousal,[12] or by light in the visual field.[13] Not all learning-disabled children with depressed PRN exhibit increases in nystagmus following SIT,[9] indicating, possibly, that for these children other forms of intervention may be warranted. It is important that therapists be able to predict which clients will be receptive to specific interventions so that the most appropriate therapy be introduced as early as possible. Ottenbacher, Short, and Watson have demonstrated that, by combining global measures of vestibular-proprioceptive and postural responding with the SCPNT, therapists are able to enhance their diagnostic procedures with learning-disabled children.[8,9]

PRN has been investigated primarily in samples of school-age children,[7,14] and published norms do not exist for large samples of preschool children. Recently, in an investigation of the test-retest reliability of the duration of SCPNT scores in 3 and 4 year olds, norms were reported for 28 and 42 subjects, respectively.[15] The authors of that study concluded that "Since the study was supportive of acceptable test-retest reliability for four-year-olds, additional reliability, validity and normative studies with this age group should be undertaken." (p 175)

Although it has been suggested[16] that "soft" neurological signs are more evident at earlier ages and become progressively more difficult to obtain, these signs have not been extensively examined in pre-school children. It might be expected that clinical assessment of vestibular and proprioceptive functions may be easier to obtain with a younger population. In addition, it is not known what relationships exist between these clinical assessment variables when they are obtained from a pre-school population. Using measures of postural control, reflex integration, and bilateral motor integration, DeGangi, Berk, and Larsen[17] reported that these vestibular-based measures showed strong discriminative ability for separating normal and delayed pre-school children. The primary purpose of the present study was to examine 4-year-old Head Start children's performance abilities on assessments of vestibular and proprioceptive functions —that is, muscle tone, various postures, balance, and PRN. A second objective was to obtain normative data for these measures and to explore the nature of the relationship between these variables and PRN within a subject sample of 4 year olds.

METHOD

Subjects. As part of the regularly scheduled screening procedures for all 4-year-old children participating in the Chattanooga area Head Start Programs, 177 four-year-old children were evaluated by one of two occupational therapists experienced in pediatric therapy. Eliminated from the sample were any children who were extremely passive or uncooperative, who refused the testing or could not remain seated on the nystagmus board, who exhibited strabismus, or who had received previous diagnoses of mental retardation or neurological disorders. As a result, the total number of subjects consisted of 156 children, 72 males and 84 females, of Black and Caucasian races, from rural and urban environments, and ranging in age from 47 to 60 months.

Procedure. In a quiet section of the children's classroom or in a separate room, clinical assessments of muscle-tone; co-contraction; prone-extension posture; supine flexion posture; one foot, standing balance-eyes open; one foot, standing balance-eyes closed; asymmetrical tonic neck relfex, and postrotary nystagmus were conducted. Standing balance was assessed according to the instructions in the Southern California Sensory Integration Tests (SCSIT);[18] nystagmus was assessed according to the standardized instructions of the SCPNT;[7] and the other five assessments were modified from those reported by Ottenbacher.[8] Modifications of the five assessments were conducted in order to increase the objectivity of assessment and scoring and to enhance communication with younger subjects. The instructions and modifications are included for comparison with Ottenbacher's methods. (It should be noted that, after this study was conducted, Dunn published *A Guide to Testing Clinical Observations in Kindergartners.*[19] This guide incorporates clear instructions, illustrations of positions, criteria for scoring, and normative data for clinical assessments including the five measures modified for this study.)

Muscle Tone (MT). Using a goniometer, the degree of flexion (measured as a negative number) or hyperextension (measured as a positive number) of the elbows is gauged. While seated in a child's chair, the child is assessed with both arms relaxed and at his or her sides. Each arm is passively extended by the therapist and scores are obtained for the right side (MT-R), and for the left side (MT-L), and a combined score (MT) is determined.

Muscle Co-Contraction (CO). The therapist and child sit facing one another. The child is instructed: "Hold onto my thumbs and keep your elbows straight." (The child's thumbs and elbows are touched and pointed out to him or her.) A practice trial is given, and, if the child flexes and extends the elbows, he or she is shown how to hold the elbows straight without locking them: "Don't bend your elbows. Now don't let me push you or pull you. Keep your arms straight." Scoring is a 1: elbows straight without locking them; 2: elbows show some flexion (5-30°) when alternately pushed and pulled; 3: elbows flex noticeably (35° or more) upon alternate pushing and pulling. If a child locks elbows in extension, he or she is shown how to relax the elbows and is given a second trial. If he or she still locks the elbows, a 3 is scored.

Prone Extension Posture (PEP). The child is asked to lie down and fly like a bird. (The child may be placed in position or it may be demonstrated.) The position is hyperextended posture with legs and arms abducted, elbows flexed, and head held above the supporting surface. The child and therapist count to see how long the child can maintain the posture—up to 20 seconds. The score is the duration (in seconds) the posture is held without having the head, arms, or knees touch the surface.

Asymmetrical Tonic Neck Reflex (ATNR). The child is asked to get on his or her hands and knees, "like a dog." (The child may be placed in position, or it may be demonstrated.) The position is quadruped. The therapist turns the child's head to the right and to the left, and observes the amount of elbow flexion as the head is turned. The head is not held in passive rotation at the end of the range, but the response is scored as the head is passively rotated toward the end of the range. A score is obtained for elbow flexion to the right (ATNR-R) and to the left (ATNR-L) as well as a combined score ATNR. A score of 1 is given if there is no flexion; 2, if there is slight flexion to 30°; 3, if there is pronounced flexion over 35°. Combined scores range from 2 to 6.

Supine Flexion Posture (SFP). The child is asked to roll up in a ball. (The child may be placed in position, or it may be demonstrated.) The position is flexion posture with arms crossed on chest, ankles crossed, and neck, hips, and knees flexed. The child and therapist count to see how long the child can maintain the posture—up to 20 seconds. The score is the duration, in seconds, the posture is held without having the legs, neck, or arms touch the surface or without breaking the symmetrical flexion posture, for example, if the child starts extending a leg, the neck, or the arms.

Standing Balance—Eyes Open (SBO). The child is asked or shown how to stand with the arms folded across the chest. As in SCSIT procedures, touching the child's left leg, the therapist asks the child to lift the foot and to keep still, not to hop or move around. The score is the duration in seconds the child holds the foot up without unfolding the arms, moving the standing foot, or touching the other foot to the ground. Score is only counted if the child maintains an erect posture and does not rest the lifted foot against the other leg. If a child does not understand, the knee is bent and placed in position as a demonstration. Instructions are repeated for lifting the right foot. Scores are obtained for the right leg (SBO-R), the left leg (SBO-L), and combined (SBO).

Standing Balance—Eyes Closed (SBC). This is conducted the same as SBO except that the child keeps the eyes closed. The duration in seconds for maintaining the posture with the right leg (SBC-R), the left leg (SBC-L), and both legs (SBC) is recorded.

Postrotary Nystagmus (PRN). This is administered according to standardized instructions in the SCPNT. Scores are obtained for the duration of PRN to the right (PRN-R), after rotation to the left (PRN-L), and combined (PRN).

The clinical assessments were administered in the order they are presented above and took between 10 and 20 minutes per child. Scores were recorded on a separate score sheet developed for this study. Although interobserver reliability scores were not obtained throughout data collection, the therapists worked closely developing high levels of agreement on all items before assessing the sample for this study. Both therapists were experienced with the clinical observations from the SCSIT,[18] from which Ottenbacher's[8] assessments were obtained. One therapist had learned the criteria from Ottenbacher and taught those criteria to the second therapist. The score sheet for testing included space for comments; if a child responded in an idiosyncratic manner, this response was recorded.

Results. Because of occasional missing data points, the sample sizes vary for the normative data. This is noted in Table 1 where sample sizes vary from 152 to 156. Because of the nature of the computer program,[20] the multiple regression analysis as well was conducted only for subjects for whom all data points were complete; therefore, the sample size for the regression was 145.

The normative data including means, standard deviations, and ranges for all of the clinical assessments except PRN are included in Table 1.

Table 1
Norms for Clinical Assessments of 4 Year Olds

Assessments		Mean	Standard Deviation	Range	No. Subjects
CO*	(score 1,2,3)	1.34	.57	1 to 3	156
MT-L	degrees (- ✔ ; + /)	2.97	5.00	-10 to +20	155
MT-R	degrees (- ✔ ; + /)	3.75	4.67	- 8 to +22	155
MT	degrees (- ✔ ; + /)	6.7	9.08	-17 to +37	155
PEP	seconds (0 - 20)	5.5	7.36	0 to 20	152
SFP	seconds (0 - 20)	14.3	6.07	0 to 20	155
ATNR-L	(1,2,3)	1.76	.73	1 to 3	153
ATNR-R	(1,2,3)	1.9	.76	1 to 3	150
ATNR	(2 - 6)	3.7	2.5	2 to 6	146
SBO-L	seconds (0 - 30)	6.69	5.84	0 to 24	156
SBO-R	seconds (0 - 30)	6.87	5.92	0 to 30	156
SBO	seconds (0 - 60)	13.56	10.10	0 to 40	156
SBC-L	seconds (0 - 30)	2.10	1.97	0 to 14	156
SBC-R	seconds (0 - 30)	2.01	2.21	0 to 14	156
SBC	seconds (0 - 60)	4.1	3.85	0 to 28	156

*See text for explanation of abbreviations for clinical assessments

These data are reported for combined scores as well as, where possible, for bilateral responses. The data for SCPNT are reported in Table 2 and also include a breakdown of scores based on sex and right and left responses.

Because Ayres[7] and Kimball[14] found discrepant results in the sex differences in the variances of PRN for 5 to 9 year olds, a test for difference between variances[21] was conducted for this study. The results indicated no significant differences between the PRN variances of the males and females ($F = 1.34$, $df = 71/83$, $p > .05$). In addition, a one-way Analysis of Variance, with sex as the independent variable and nystagmus as the dependent variable, indicated no significant differences between the males and females in their PRN responses ($F = .01$, $df = 1/155$, $p > .9$).

Using PRN as the dependent variable and MT, ATNR, CO, PEP, SFP, SBO, SBC, and sex as independent variables, a step-wise multiple regression[14] was used to determine the relationship of the independent variables in predicting PRN. The single best predictor was CO, but this only accounted for 7 percent of the variance of PRN. The remaining variables, in order of amount of contribution to the prediction of PRN are: PEP, FSP, ATNR, SBO, sex, and MT. SBC contributed so little that it was not included in the regression. Together the variables only accounted for 13.5 percent of the variance of PRN. The cumulative regression R-squares as well as simple rs, showing the correlation of nystagmus with each of these variables, are included in Table 3.

Because of the recent findings that clinical variables may be better predictors of PRN for children who exhibit depressed nystagmus,[9] an additional regression was conducted using the same independent variables to predict PRN. This was conducted, however, only for subjects who scored lower than 1 standard deviation below the mean on the SCPNT. Twenty-eight subjects evidenced nystagmus of 6 seconds or less; however, because of missing data points, the regression analysis was performed on 25 children.

Table 2
Norms for Duration of Postrotary Nystagmus in 4-Year-Old Children

Assessment	Mean	Standard Deviation	Range	No. of Subjects
Combined Males and Females				
PRN-Left	9.08	6.12	0-34	156
PRN-Right	9.28	6.75	0-40	156
PRN-Total	18.34	11.95	0-60	156
Females				
PRN-Left	9.24	5.42	0-27	81
PRN-Right	9.23	6.63	0-27	81
PRN-Total	18.46	11.15	0-54	81
Males				
PRN-Left	8.9	6.89	0-34	72
PRN-Right	9.3	6.94	0-40	72
PRN-Total	18.2	12.89	0-60	72

Table 3
Relation Between Postrotary Nystagmus and Clinical Assessments in 4-Year-Old Children*

	Regression R-Square	Correlation Coefficient (Simple r)
CO	.07	.27
PEP	.04	.17
SFP	.02	-.13
ATNR	.01	-.14
SBO	.001	-.06
SEX	.0005	-.005
MT	.0002	.01
Cumulative total	.135	

*N = 145

For these subjects, the independent variables, in order of contribution to the regression, are PEP, SBO, MT, sex, SFP, CO, and ATNR. PEP was the best predictor, accounting for 12 percent of the variance; PEP, SBO, and MT together accounted for 37 percent of the variance of PRN, and all of the variables accounted for 50 percent. The cumulative regression R-squares and simple rs are included in Table 4.

DISCUSSION

A large quantity of data was generated in this study. The normative data for all of the clinical assessments may be useful for other therapists using such evaluations with other preschool populations. Some of the tasks, notably PEP and SBC, were difficult for the 4-year-old children. For example, the mean SBC score was 4.1 seconds compared with the mean of SBO, which was 13.56 seconds. The mean PEP score was 5.5 seconds compared with SFP, which was 14.3 seconds. Dunn's[19] assessments of 5-year-old children are similar. She reports that "It seems reasonable to expect five-year-olds to execute the supine flexion posture and hold it without resistance for a period of time." (p21) However, on the prone extension posture with legs straight, "many children exhibited so short a duration performance that it would be difficult to separate normal children who could not maintain the posture very long from children with difficulty.'' (p 24) This is in contrast with Harris'[22] report of mean scores of 18.15 seconds for 4-year-olds' performance on prone extension. One possible explanation for this difference is that the present study and Dunn's guide (in position #3) required the child to extend at the hips, keeping the knees straight, and maintaining the knees off the supporting surface. It is not clear whether Harris maintained this strict criterion. Many children in the present study could have assumed and maintained the PEP posture for much longer if the leg extension criterion had not been included. Dunn[19] confirms this. Looking at four different extension postures, she reported that the three that required leg extension, with the legs off the floor, were very difficult for kindergarten children. Another possible explanation for the difference between the PEP scores in the present study and Harris' scores is the difference in duration of holding the posture. The present study stopped at 20 seconds, whereas Harris continued to 30 seconds. It is possible that a ceiling effect in this study caused the mean to be much lower than Harris's. This is a doubtful explanation, however, because only 19 children in the present study were able to maintain the posture for 20 seconds, compared with at least 3 times that number who could not even assume the posture.

The nystagmus duration scores for the males and females combined in

Table 4
Relation Between Postrotary Nystagmus and Clinical Assessments in 4-Year-Old Children with Low Nystagmus*

	Regression R-Square	Correlation Coefficient (Simple r)
PEP	.12	.35
SBO	.12	.34
MT	.13	-.17
SEX	.03	.16
SFP	.02	.34
SBC	.03	.31
CO	.04	.28
ATNR	.001	.07
Cumulative total	.498	

*Less than one standard deviation below the mean; N = 25

this study are similar to those combined scores for 4 year olds examined by Deitz, Siegner, and Crowe.[15] Their initial SCPNT duration mean was 19.57 seconds compared with their re-test score of 18.93 seconds, and compared with 18.34 seconds in this study. The data are more variable, however, when they are separated by sex. In the study by Deitz et al., the mean total SCPNT duration for males (initial: 21.87 sec, re-test: 20.87 sec) and females (initial: 16.79 sec, retest: 16.58 sec) differs by 4-5 seconds. In the present study, the mean scores for the males (18.2 sec) and females (18.46) do not differ but are less than the scores for males and greater than the scores for females reported by Deitz et al. It is not reported whether Deitz et al., found significant sex differences, but of the 5- to 9-year-olds investigated by Ayres,[7] significant sex differences between the variances of the SCPNT duration scores necessitated the development of separate standardization data for each sex. Kimball[14] and the present study reported no such significant sex differences.

Another difference between all of these studies is variability. In Ayres' manual of normative data for SCPNT scores for 5 to 9 year olds, no subjects received a total score of zero; and the maximum longest duration was 24 seconds.[7] In the present study, 7 males and 4 females exhibited nystagmus durations of zero; and the maximum PRN duration in one direction was 40 seconds. Obviously, this sample is more variable, with a combined (male-female, right-left) standard deviation of 11.9 seconds, compared with Ayres' 7 seconds, Kimball's 9.67 seconds, and 6.87 seconds reported by Deitz et al. Kimball has discussed the implications of interpreting PRN data with higher variability; essentially, it causes an increased range of scores that are considered to be within normal limits and increases, especially the cut-off point for determining whether a score is deviantly high. Because her data were more variable than those reported by Ayres,[7] Kimball has suggested that there may be regional differences in the norms for PRN and that this needs to be further examined.[14] The present study presents similar problems because of high variability, which could, in part, be due to lack of interobserver reliability. It should be pointed out that both Ayres'[7] and Kimball's[14] data were obtained from middle class, non-Black populations. Deitz et al., do not specify the racial or economic background of their sample, which comes from a metropolitan area in the state of Washington. The present study was conducted with a lower class, mixed race, Southern, combined urban and rural population. Whether the causes for such differences in variability between studies is due to sample characteristics such as geographic, racial, or economic background or other factors needs further exploration. In addition, the reasons for discrepancies in sex differences between studies will require further experimental analysis.

Ottenbacher[8] reported that the variables PEP, SBC, MT, and SBO share significant variance with SCPNT scores obtained in school-aged children diagnosed with learning disabilities, minimal brain dysfunction, or perceptual motor disabilities. The present study, using the same clinical assessments, was able to account for only 13.5 percent of the variance of SCPNT scores in normal Head Start 4-year-old children. This suggests that these variables may not be clinically useful for screening normal 4 year olds for possible manifestation of vestibular deficits. That these variables are useful, however, for subdividing populations of children already diagnosed as learning disabled has been demonstrated.[9] Thus, the measures of balance, tone, and extension posture may show better predictive relationships in children with depressed nystagmus. In the present study, PEP, SBO, MT, sex, SFP, SBC, CO, and ATNR (in that order) accounted for 50 percent of the variance of SCPNT scores that were less than 1 standard deviation below the mean. Clyse[23] has demonstrated that a measure of dynamic balance may be an even better indicator of vestibular dysfunction than standing balance. She reported that the walk-on-floor-eyes-closed test of the Floor Ataxia Test Battery,[24] a measure of dynamic balance, in combination with PEP, accounted for 50 percent of the variance of SCPNT scores in school-aged children with learning disabilities or perceptual motor dysfunction.

In the present study, in the sample of children with depressed nystagmus, the variable muscle tone shows an inverse correlation with SCPNT. This means that, as the score on tone increases, nystagmus decreases. With the method of assessing muscle tone for this particular study, hyperextension is a positive score so that these data are consistent with Ottenbacher's[8] report that low nystagmus is correlated with hypotonia. Whether the muscle tone assessment used in this study is an adequate and accurate reflection of tone is questionable. However, using this particular measure makes it possible to compare with Ottenbacher's previous studies[8,9] and provides a quantitative measure. In her clinical assessment of tone, Dunn[19] also measures hyperextensibility of the elbow joint; however, in addition, she includes a measure of palpation. Dunn reports that "clinical impressions from palpation of muscles may be more helpful than measurement of the elbow joint in determining the integrity of muscle tone." (p 8) The problem with using palpation as a variable is that it is difficult to objectify and quantify.

Implications for Occupational Therapy. The study of learning disabilities in pre-school populations is particularly difficult. These children have not yet acquired many of the fine, perceptual-motor, academic abilities that are used to gauge learning disabilities in older children. Therefore, clinical observations of tone, reflex integration, posture, and postrotary nystagmus, which are useful for indicating vestibular-processing deficits in school-age learning-disabled children[9,23] may also be useful for discriminating delayed pre-school children.[17] Standardized assessments and norms for these sensorimotor abilities are limited,[17] although the present study and other recent investigations have contributed information on the performance of pre-school children on postrotary nystagmus,[15] prone extension posture,[22] and many other clinical observations.[19] The results of the present study suggest that, in contrast to their use with school-age learning-disabled children, clinical measures of tone, balance, and extension posture are not good predictors of depressed nystagmus in a large group of normal pre-school Head Start children. It is suggested, as it has been with older learning-disabled children[8,9,23] that, if therapists use clinical measures to predict possible vestibular deficits, they include a constellation of measures along with SCPNT scores. This shows the need for normative measures of all clinical variables including SCPNT scores for 3, 4, and 5 year olds. The study by Deitz et al.[15] and the present study provide some norms; however, due to sex differences, and possible racial or regional differences,[7,14] it is advisable that more normative data be acquired in order to present a clear profile of the SCPNT scores of preschool children.[15] Therapists should also be cautious in generalizing the data from this study because of the lack of interobserver reliability determination throughout the study and because Head Start children may not be representative of all preschool children. These data can be used, in combination with other normative measures, as guides for performance skills.

The results from this and from Dunn's guide[19] suggest that some clinical measures are not particularly useful for pre-school children. The skills of one-leg-standing-balance—eyes closed, and prone extension posture with legs extended off the supporting surface, are very difficult for 4-year-old and kindergarten children[19] and therefore may not be useful assessment criteria. The regression analyses from this study suggest that continued research needs to be conducted into the relationship between clinical observations and vestibular functions in pre-school children.

REFERENCES

1. Hayden AH, Smith RK, von Kippel CS, Baer SA: *Mainstreaming Preschoolers: Children with Learning Disabilities* (DHEW Publication No. OHOS, 78-31117). Washington, DC: US Government Printing Office, 1978

2. Lahey BB, Hobbs SA, Kupfer DL, Delamater A: Current perspectives on hyperactivity and learning disabilities. In *Behavior Therapy with Hyperactive and Learning Disabled Children*, B. Lahey, Editor. New York: Oxford University Press, 1979

3. Wender PH: The minimal brain dysfunction syndrome in children. *J Nerv Ment Dis* 153:55-71, 1972

4. Ayres AJ: Deficits in sensory integration in educationally handicapped children. *J Learn Disabil* 2: 160-168, 1969

5. Saunders TR: A critical analysis of the minimal brain dysfunction syndrome. *Prof Psychol* 10: 293-306, 1979

6. deQuiros JB, Schrager O: *Neuropsychological Fundamentals in Learning Disabilities,* San Rafael, CA: Academic Therapy, 1978

7. Ayres AJ: *Southern California Postrotary Nystagmus Test: Manual,* Los Angeles: Western Psychological Services, 1975

8. Ottenbacher K: Identifying vestibular processing dysfunction in learning-disabled children. *Am J Occup Ther* 32: 217-221, 1978

9. Ottenbacher K, Short MA, Watson, PJ: The use of selected clinical observations to predict postrotary nystagmus change in learning disabled children. *Phys Occup Ther Ped* 1: 31-38, 1980

10. Ayres AJ: *Sensory Integration and Learning Disorders,* Los Angeles: Western Psychological Services, 1972

11. Ayres AJ: Learning disabilities and the vestibular system. *J Learn Disabil* 11: 30-40, 1978

12. Cogan D: *Neurology of the Ocular Muscles* (2nd Edition), Springfield, IL: Charles C Thomas, 1956

13. Levy D, Proctor L, Holzman P: Visual interference on vestibular response. *Arch Otolaryngol* 103: 287-291, 1977

14. Kimball JG: Normative comparison of the Southern California Postrotary Nystagmus Test: Los Angeles vs. Syracuse data. *Am J Occup Ther* 35: 21-25, 1981

15. Deitz J, Seigner C, Crowe T: The Southern California Postrotary Nystagmus Test: Test-retest reliability for preschool children. *Occup Ther J Res* 1: 165-177, 1981

16. Frank J, Levinson H: Dysmetric dyslexia and dyspraxia. *Acad Ther* 11: 133-143, 1975-76

17. DeGangi GA, Berk RA, Larsen LA: The measurement of vestibular-based functions in preschool children. *Am J Occup Ther* 34: 452-459, 1980

18. Ayres AJ: *Southern California Sensory Integration Tests,* Los Angeles: Western Psychological Services, 1972

19. Dunn W: *A Guide to Testing Clinical Observations in Kindergartners,* Rockville, MD The American Occupational Therapy Association, 1981

20. Nie NH, Hull CH, Jenkins JG, Steinbrenner K, Bent DH: *Statistical Package for the Social Sciences,* New York: McGraw-Hill, 1975

21. Bruning JL, Kintz BL: *Computational Handbook of Statistics* (2nd Edition). Dallas, TX: Scott, Foresman and Co., 1977

22. Harris NP: Duration and quality of the prone extension position in four-, six-, and eight-year-old normal children, *Am J Occup Ther* 35: 26-30, 1981

23. Clyse S: Dynamic balance and vestibular function in the learning disabled. Unpublished master's thesis, Boston University, 1981

24. Fregly AR, Graybiel A: An ataxia test battery not requiring rails. *Aerospace Med* 39: 277-281, 1968

The Relationship Between Dynamic Balance and Postrotary Nystagmus in Learning-Disabled Children

Sally J. Clyse
Margaret A. Short

ABSTRACT. Twenty-four children with learning disabilities or perceptual-motor handicaps were evaluated using the Southern California Postrotary Nystagmus Test and other clinical measures frequently used by occupational therapists to assess vestibular function. Correlational analyses revealed significant relationships between nystagmus duration scores and Walk on Floor Eyes Closed (a test of dynamic balance), prone extension posture, Walk on Floor Eyes Open, age, muscle tone and Standing Balance: Eyes Open. Multiple regression analysis indicated that when all of the clinical variables were considered together, the Walk on Floor Eyes Closed test was the best predictor of postrotary nystagmus duration. These findings expand the results of other studies which have related clinical vestibular tests to duration of postrotary nystagmus and also indicate that therapists may want to include assessments of dynamic balance with other clinical variables in the evaluation of vestibular function.

A wide range of clinical disorders have been found in learning disabled children. Many of these disorders have been shown to comprise syndromes associated with vestibular-proprioceptive deficits.[1-4] One of these syndromes, originally identified by Ayres as a disorder in postural and bilateral integration, was characterized by poorly integrated postural mechanisms, muscle hypotonia, poor equilibrium reactions and poor ocular control.[5] The subsequent development of the Southern California Sensory Integration Tests (SCSIT)[1] and the Southern California Postrotary Nystagmus Test (SCPNT)[6] provided clinicians with assessments to further elaborate vestibular-proprioceptive disorders. Ottenbacher,[3] however, suggested that in order for therapists to obtain a clear profile of vestibular deficits, they should not rely on one evaluation, e.g., SCPNT scores, but should include a constellation of variables. This is supported by Montgomery and Capps, who reported that nystagmus responses were affected by arousal levels in normal children. These authors were concerned that therapists may wrongly attribute abnormal nystagmus responses, "directly to the vestibular system when the cause may be due to other central nervous system mechanisms'';[7(p.27)] and they recommended that ''therapists involved in evaluative procedures use a wide range of test scores and clinical observations before determining that a child has a vestibular-based problem.''[7(p. 27)]

The purpose of the present study was to expand our knowledge of the relationship among clinical variables that have been linked to vestibular-proprioceptive dysfunction. Using a number of these clinical measures, Ottenbacher reported that, in learning disabled children, performance on prone extension posture, standing balance eyes closed (SBC), muscle tone, and standing balance eyes open (SBO), (in that order) were the best predictors of SCPNT duration scores.[3] Both Ottenbacher and Ayres have linked a static measure of balance, i.e., maintaining equilibrium for one position of the body as in standing on one foot, to vestibular function. Dynamic balance, however, which involves maintaining equilibrium while the body is in motion, may present an even greater challenge to the vestibular system than static balance and may, therefore, be more useful as an assessment variable.

Previous studies have demonstrated the use of dynamic balance assessment in subjects with vestibular dysfunction. For example, measures of tandem walking, which assess dynamic balance, have been used to identify adults with vestibular dysfunction.[8] Using the Floor Ataxia Test Battery, Fregly and Graybiel[9] demonstrated that vestibular-defective subjects were unable to walk heel to toe in a straight line when their eyes were closed but were able to perform this task when their eyes were open. The same subjects were able to perform tasks that measured static balance (e.g., standing on both feet with eyes closed, or standing on one foot with eyes open). Birren[10] also described a vestibular-impaired patient who was able to perform normally on static balance tasks but was unable to perform a dynamic balance task. This loss of dynamic balance in the presence of intact static balance suggests the better discriminatory power of dynamic balance measures over those of static balance in predicting vestibular deficits.

As a result, the present study was designed to determine if dynamic balance is an important variable to include in the clinical evaluation of vestibular functioning. This study was also designed to extend Ottenbacher's[3] findings that prone extension posture, SBC, muscle tone and SBO are predictors of SCPNT scores in learning disabled children. The following two hypotheses were tested: 1) a significant positive correlation would be found between performance on the Walk on Floor Eyes Closed (WOFEC) tandem walking test from the Floor Ataxia Test Battery[9] and performance on the SCPNT in children with learning disabilities or perceptual-motor handicaps, and 2) the dynamic balance measures, WOFEC and WOFEO would be better predictors of PRN duration than would the static balance measures, SBC and SBO.

METHOD

Subjects

Twenty-nine public school children participated in the study, however, only twenty-four completed testing. Subjects came from a variety of socio-economic backgrounds, residing in cities and towns in the North Shore of Boston. All subjects were considered to have a learning disability or perceptual-motor handicap by the occupational therapist or teacher working with them. School reports indicated that all subjects were within the normal range of intelligence. Subjects with overt physical handicaps such as blindness, deafness, or cerebral palsy were excluded from the study. Five subjects were omitted from the final data analysis because they refused or were unable to complete the SCPNT. The twenty-four remaining subjects were eight females and sixteen males ranging in ages from 76-118 months, with a combined mean age of 94.8 months.

Procedure

Each subject was individually tested on seven variables by one of two occupational therapists. Interrater reliabilities were obtained on each of the seven variables by simultaneous testing of six subjects two weeks prior to data collection. The methods and scoring criteria which were used for each variable are described; following a description of each variable are the interrater reliability coefficient (r), mean ($\bar{x}$) and standard deviation (SD) for each test.

Standing Balance: Eyes Open (SBO)—According to the Standing Balance: Eyes Open test of the SCSIT[1]—Scoring was according to the standardized instructions in the test manual with the following exceptions: 1) after the subject had stood for 60 seconds the test was stopped for that foot; 2) the subjects were not allowed to hook the lifted foot behind the knee of the supporting leg; and 3) the best performance out of two trials constituted the score unless the maximum score of 60 was met on the first trial. The combined right and left raw score was used for analysis. (r = +.99; $\bar{x}$ = 42.67; SD = 31.53)

Standing Balance: Eyes Closed (SBC)—According to the Standing Balance: Eyes Closed test of the SCSIT[1]—the same exceptions in scoring as noted in SBO applied. (r = +.98; $\bar{x}$ = 9.04; SD = 5.75)

Walk On Floor Eyes Open (WOFEO)—According to the Walk on Floor Eyes Open test of the Floor Ataxia Test Battery[9]—This test consisted of walking as straight as possible ten heel-to-toe steps beyond the first two starting steps with arms folded against chest. A maximum of five trials were administered. The best three out of five trials constituted the score. The maximum test score obtainable was 30 (10 steps × 3 trials).

Trials during which the foot position was violated either by nontandem alignment of feet or by toe not touching heel were terminated. (r = +.97; x̄ = 21.62; SD = 8.69)

Walk On Floor Eyes Closed (WOFEC)—According to the Walk On Floor Eyes Closed test of the Floor Ataxia Test Battery.[9] This test was administered and scored the same as WOFEO with the exception that the eyes were closed. (r = +.90; x̄ = 5.87; SD = 6.66)

Prone Extension Posture (PEP)—As described by Ottenbacher[3]—The subject was asked to lie prone and maintain a hyperextended posture with legs, arms and head held above the supporting surface. As opposed to Ottenbacher's three point scale, the score was the duration in seconds the posture was held without having the head, arms or knees touch the surface. The child was either placed in this position or the position was demonstrated to him. A stopwatch was used for timing. (r = +.99; x̄ = 19.45; SD = 10.83)

Muscle Tone (MT)—As described by Ottenbacher[3]—the degree of muscle tone was evaluated by passively extending the joints of the upper extremities. Scoring was based on a 3-point scale, with 1 definite hypotonicity, 2 slight hypotonicity, and 3 normal. (r = +.94; x̄ = 2.00; SD = 0.72)

Southern California Postrotary Nystagmus Test (SCPNT)—According to standardized instructions in the SCPNT[6] manual. Total raw scores in seconds were used for analysis. (r = +.94; x̄ = 16.91; SD = 5.80)

RESULTS

As indicated by the correlation results in Table 1, WOFEC was significantly positively correlated with SCPNT as were the variables prone extension posture, WOFEO, age, muscle tone and SBO. That is, as nystagmus duration scores decreased, scores on all other variables decreased as well. Stepwise multiple regression was employed to determine which of the independent variables shared the most variance, i.e., was the best predictor of the dependent variable, SCPNT. As illustrated in Table 2, WOFEC was determined to be the best predictor, explaining 30% of the variance in SCPNT scores. Table 2 lists the R^2 values for each of the remaining independent variables. (The R^2 value is the amount of variance in the dependent variable which is explained by each independent variable.) As Table 2 illustrates, the additional variables (in order of greatest shared variance with SCPNT) were prone extension posture, muscle tone, WOFEO, age and SBC. Of importance is the fact that WOFEC and prone extension posture, considered together, explained 52% of the variance in SCPNT, while the remaining variables explained only an additional 8%. Standing Balance: Eyes Open is reported as zero in Table 2 because it contributed an insignificant amount of variance.

Table 1

Correlation[+] of Clinical Variables with SCPNT

	WOFEC[++]	PEP	WOFEO	AGE	MT	SBO	SBC
SCPNT	.55****	.53***	.50***	.41**	.41**	.37*	.31

+ Pearson Product Moment Correlation Coefficient

++ see text for explanation of abbreviations

$p \leq .05*$, .025**, .01***, .005****, (df/24)

Table 2

Multiple Regression R - Square Values

Independent Variables

		WOFEC	PEP	MT	WOFEO	AGE	SBC	SBO
Dependent Variable	SCPNT	.30	.22	.04	.03	.01	.001	.00
	CUMULATIVE R-SQUARE	.30	.52	.56	.59	.60	.601	.601

DISCUSSION

This study demonstrated that as the duration of PRN decreased in children with learning disabilities or perceptual-motor handicaps, the performance on WOFEC, a dynamic balance test, declined as well. In addition, the dynamic balance measures, WOFEC and WOFEO were shown to be more rigorous predictors of PRN duration, than were the static balance measures, SBC and SBO. The results of this study indicate that dynamic balance-eyes closed, as measured by the WOFEC test, is an important variable to include in the evaluation of vestibular function in learning disabled children. In addition, these findings support earlier research that showed a relationship between depressed performance on dynamic balance eyes closed, as measured by the WOFEC test, and vestibular impairment in adults.[8] The findings of this present study also agree, in general, with the conclusions of Ottenbacher.[3] He reported that prone extension posture, SBC and muscle tone are related to PRN in learning disabled children. In this study, SBO did not share significant variance with SCPNT as it did in Ottenbacher's study, but this may be the result of the inclusion of the dynamic balance assessments which provide a greater challenge to the vestibular system than does SBO.

The results of this study suggest that, in addition to the variables outlined by Ottenbacher and Ayres,[3,5] dynamic balance as measured by WOFEC may be a critical variable to include in the clinical evaluation of vestibular function. Because its administration is simple, the WOFEC test is well suited for use by occupational and physical therapists when evaluating vestibular function in learning disabled children. The WOFEC test takes approximately five minutes to administer and requires only a stopwatch. Normative data for the WOFEC are available for male and female children at age levels 8, 10, 12, 14, 16, and 18 years;[11] and it has been validated as a standardized test for identifying adults with vestibular function.[8,9] As Cunningham and Goetzinger point out, however, the validity of this test with children cannot be determined "until a group of labyrinthine-defective children and children with other equilibrium defects can be tested."[11(p. 564)]

Therapists must realize that many different methods exist for assessing vestibular function. DeQuiros and Schrager have divided tests of vestibular function into otological and clinical categories. Among the otological assessments are caloric tests, which involve irrigating the external ear canal with cold or warm water; rotary tests, which consist of turning movements e.g., in a swivel chair like the Barany's test, or on a rotary board like the SCPNT; and linear acceleration tests, used primarily for assessing newborns. All of these otological tests provide information regarding labyrinthine function by examining nystagmus responses.[12]

The clinical tests, on the other hand, examine posture, equilibrium, and muscle tone. These would include the WOFEO, WOFEC and other assessments of dynamic balance as well as assessment of prone extension posture, muscle tone and standing balance. Although many of these assessments are currently being used by occupational and physical therapists, the nature of the relationships among all of these different variables has only begun to be explored. For example, Ottenbacher, Short and Watson have demonstrated that the four variables, prone extension posture, SBC, muscle tone, and SBO can collectively be used to predict which low nystagmus learning disabled children will respond with increases in nystagmus duration after exposure to sensory integration therapy.[13] The value of using clinical variables for predicting which children may most benefit from specific forms of therapy is obvious. The results of the present study suggest that assessment of dynamic balance would contribute to this predictive efficacy. In addition, clinical research would be advanced by the further exploration of relationships between performance of learning disabled children on the WOFEC test and performance on otological tests, other than the SCPNT, such as caloric or linear acceleration tests. The work of Montgomery and Capps[7] has suggested a number of investigations aimed at the exploration of relationships between clinical variables while controlling for or accounting for the effects of arousal on nystagmus measures; such research should enhance our diagnostic success. The conclusions of Montgomery and Capps[7] and Ottenbacher[3] suggest that, because the reliability of the assessment of a single variable is limited, diagnosis of a vestibular disorder should include evaluation of a group of variables. The present study suggests that dynamic balance be one of them.

REFERENCES

1. Ayres AJ: *Southern California Sensory Integration Tests*. Los Angeles, Western Psychological Services, 1972.

2. DeQuiros J: Diagnosis of vestibular disorders in the learning disabled. *J Learn Disabil* 9: 50-58, 1976.

3. Ottenbacher K: Identifying vestibular processing dysfunction in learning disabled children. *Am J Occup Ther* 32: 217-221, 1978.

4. Steinberg M, Rendle-Short J: Vestibular dysfunction in young children with minor neurological impairment. *Dev Med Child Neurol* 19: 639-651, 1977.

5. Ayres AJ: Characteristics of types of sensory integrative dysfunction. *Am J Occup Ther* 25: 329-334, 1971.

6. Ayres AJ: *Southern California Postrotary Nystagmus Test*. Los Angeles, Western Psychological Services, 1975.

7. Montgomery P, Capps MJ: Effects of arousal on the nystagmus response of normal children. *Phys Occup Ther Pediatr* 1:17-29, 1980.

8. Fregly AR, Graybiel A: Labrinthine defects as shown by ataxia and caloric tests, *Acta Otolaryngol* 69:216-222, 1970.

9. Fregly AR, Graybiel A: An ataxia test battery not requiring rails. *Aerospace Med* 39: 277-282, 1968.

10. Birren J: Static equilibrium and vestibular function. *J Exper Psychol* 35:129-133, 1945.

11. Cunningham DR, Goetzinger CP: Floor ataxia test battery. *Arch Otolaryngol* 96:559-564, 1972.

12. DeQuiros JB, Schrager O: *Neuropsychological Fundamentals in Learning Disabilities*. San Rafael, CA, Academic Therapy, 1978.

13. Ottenbacher K, Short MA, Watson PJ: The use of selected clinical observations to predict postrotary nystagmus change in learning disabled children. *Phys Occup Ther Pediatr* 1:31-38, 1980.

PART 3:
COLLABORATION AND THE ETHICS
OF RESEARCH

Most of the studies included in this anthology are the result of a collaboration between several individuals who developed a series of research questions. These questions arose from two different bases: clinical observations made during treatment of learning disabled children at the East Tennessee Children's Rehabilitation Center and predictions made from published research by Ayres,[1] DeQuiros and Schrager,[2] and others. The correlational studies discussed in Part 2 illustrate that certain clinical variables can predict postrotary nystagmus (prn). Many additional questions, however, had arisen. Observations of the children who displayed low prn seemed to indicate that they, especially, were responsive to treatment using sensory integration procedures. We wondered if we could experimentally follow their improvements by repeatedly taking certain measurements over the course of therapy. We also wondered if we could predict, based on specific clinical variables, which children would exhibit responses to therapy.

These types of predictions are very important to therapists. Clinical therapists would like to have the ability to predict which clients will respond to intervention and to measure the clients' changes over time. Ken's and Jane's clinical observations had concurred with sensory integration theory, which predicts that learning disabled children with low prn should respond to therapy with increases in nystagmus durations.[1] The purpose of the following research was to test this prediction. Additionally, we were curious about other observations we had made about this specific group of learning disabled children who exhibited low (or zero) prn. We informally observed that these children had more instances of behavioral problems when compared with other children in the clinic. We also hypothesized that since these children were learning disabled, already exhibiting ocular deficits in prn durations, perhaps one of the reasons for their learning problems could be traced to poor ocular skills.

In two studies, "Nystagmus and Ocular Fixation Difficulties in Learning-Disabled Children" (Reprint 5), and "Association between Nystagmus Hyporesponsivity and Behavioral Problems in Learning-Disabled

Children'' (Reprint 6), we explored these areas. We examined teachers' reports regarding the children's behaviors in school, and we tested the children in the clinic using a simple assessment of ocular fixation. Both studies confirmed our original "hunches" that learning disabled children with low prn exhibit more socially inappropriate behaviors and poorer ocular fixation abilities than do children with longer nystagmus durations. Both of these studies, however, had problems. A "clean" study shows a clear relationship between variables, and, unfortunately, neither of these studies is "clean". The examination of behavioral problems was complicated by sex differences, and both studies can be criticized because we created "artificial" categories by grouping together children with either low, normal, or high nystagmus responses.

CONFOUNDING VARIABLES

A further complication, which haunted us in subsequent studies, was the finding that the children with low prn tended to be younger than the children with longer nystagmus durations. Perhaps younger children who are referred to a clinic may have even greater deficits which cause them to be identified at earlier ages. Or, perhaps younger children have had less of an opportunity for therapy and are less mature. This additional variable, age, always meant that our data could be subject to multiple interpretations. For example, in the behavioral problems study, we reported that children with hyporesponsive prn displayed more behavioral problems than did a comparison group of children with higher nystagmus durations (Reprint 6). This finding *could* have been due to motor and balance-related problems causing the children to be frustrated and to act out, however, the confounding age variable offers another interpretation. Since the boys with low prn were younger, they could have been more socially inappropriate simply because of immaturity. This interpretive problem is discussed in the study; in fact the shortcomings in both studies are clearly discussed.

ETHICS OF RESEARCH

Reporting Research Problems

One of the obligations of a good researcher is to be aware of the problems of his or her research and to report those problems. No study occurs without problems, and a discussion of complications and shortcomings of a study is important for a number of reasons. For example, problems encountered during the study may actually interfere with the results, and the study may be compromised. Additionally, reporting problems may save work for the next researcher. Researchers should not be embarrassed by complications during their study; in fact some of the most exciting findings in science have been the results of errors during research. Additionally, as we explained in Part 2, conclusions drawn from a single study should always be considered tentative. Research needs to be examined within a context, and evaluations of the problems and generalizability of one particular study should be based on a framework from other related research.

Other ethical considerations regarding research involve determination of authorship, conducting research as a part of one's job, determining control groups among subjects who are participating in therapy, and obtaining permission to conduct research.

Determining Authorship

Most of the studies collected here have multiple authors. The studies reflect the contributions of a number of individuals. On many of the studies, Ken Ottenbacher is the first author. This represents the fact that he had conceptualized most of the studies, made the original observations on which the studies were based, or collected the data, or wrote the rough draft of the manuscript. The positions of the second, third, and other authors depend upon the extent of their input to the total research project. Other responsibilities included analyzing the data, writing the manuscript, and, as with most manuscripts, re-writing and re-writing. In our group of three, it was difficult to pinpoint where ideas started. Ideas are not owned, and in a dynamic collaboration, thinking ignites, and ideas spark readily and often. This particular line of research, however, had been initiated and conceptualized by Ken; thus he is the first author of many of the studies.

Research involves a lot of work beyond coming up with an idea: organizing the study, collecting data, analyzing data, writing up a rough draft, re-writing depending upon colleague feedback, writing a draft for a particular journal, re-writing depending upon editor and reviewer feedback, and perhaps re-writing again. Depending upon the extent of their input to each total research project, other authors were included and the order of authorship determined. Frequently other individuals contributed to parts of studies, and they were included as authors. For example, Mike Biderman, a psychologist at the University of Tennessee at Chattanooga, assisted with computer data analysis and interpretation. Charlotte Rogers was an occupational therapist with Head Start during one of the studies, and she helped revise the clinical assessment for preschool children and helped collect the data for one study.

Clinical research is never conducted solely by one person, as other professionals often (and should) have input, not to mention the contributions of the subjects, co-therapists, and the administration and facility where the study is conducted. Authorship should not be taken lightly, and the problems of authorship can become highly political, especially in academic "publish or perish" environments. While including someone as an author is sometimes politically expeditious, general guidelines are that authorship is assigned only to individuals directly involved in conceptualizing, designing, conducting, and completing a study. To include as an author someone who does not understand the purpose, extent, or background of the work is inappropriate. To avoid conflicts or misunderstandings when the time comes to write up a project, a research group must discuss and clearly understand who are the authors and what is their order on the final publication. Negotiating this before the investigation is begun can prevent unnecessary confusion and embarrassment at the end of the project. If two or more individuals have contributed equally and cannot determine the order of authorship, they can alternate order if they intend to publish frequently. Or they can pick names at random or alphabetically. The order of authorship does matter, especially in academic circles where the first author is generally regarded to have made the greatest contribution to the study.

Authors have a number of ways to acknowledge the assistance of individuals who have contributed to but do not deserve authorship of a study. One of the most obvious ways is to refer to influential work in the text and in the reference section of the study. Even if the work has not been published, unpublished works, workshops, and personal communications can be cited. Another way of acknowledging someone's assistance is in a footnote to the study. The footnote should include grant support, outside assistance, and any relevant personal references the authors want to include. Examples include noting that the study was developed for part of a class or a thesis, noting that parts of a manuscript had been delivered at a conference, or thanking other therapists, administrators, colleagues, or parents of subjects for assistance or guidance during the study.

Subjects' Rights

The roles of subjects and parents of subjects is critical in any study. Most facilities have ethical guidelines or committees designed to review research protocols to prevent harm to any subjects during the administration of any research project. Releases need to be obtained for all subjects who participate in a study, and special releases need to be obtained for photographs of subjects. One way to minimize the problem of obtaining release signatures in clinical research is to include a statement which the subject (or parent or custodian) signs at the time of intake evaluation. The text of such a statement typically notes that during intervention, the client would be participating in a research project, that the project would cause no harm to the client, and that the client's rights would be protected. During the study and while reporting the results of any study, every effort should be made to protect each subject's rights to privacy. Reports of subjects' performances on evaluations should be coded by number, not name. Patients should be able to terminate their participation in research projects at any time, and they should routinely be informed of this on a release statement.

Creating a Control Group in the Clinic

One of the difficulties with using experimental designs in the clinic is the determination of a control group. In well-designed experimental studies, one group receives an intervention, while a control group does not. It is considered by some to be unethical to withhold clinical treatment, thus it may be difficult to designate an "untreated" control group. One method for overcoming this problem is to offer different kinds (duration, frequency, intensity) of treatment for comparison purposes. The problem with such a method is that both forms of treatment may cause an effect, and no differences will be apparent between groups. Thus, the purpose of the study, to determine if one particular kind of therapy is effective, is defeated. Other suggestions are to offer two entirely different forms of therapy, to stagger the introduction of intervention, or to have a baseline intervention for both groups and to "add on" the treatment under investigation.

Each of these suggestions has drawbacks. One of these procedures was used in the last study in this anthology, "The Effects of a Clinically Applied Program of Vestibular Stimulation on the Neuromotor Performance of Children With Severe Developmental Disability" (Reprint 12). In this study, the intervention under investigation was vestibular stimulation. The treatment group received vestibular stimulation plus skill training, while the control group received skill training alone. The results of the study indicated that the treatment group demonstrated significant gains over the control group. Conclusions regarding these data are complicated because the gains made by the treatment group cannot be attributed solely to the effects of vestibular stimulation. Since the treatment subjects received a combination of treatments, it can only be concluded that the combination was effective. Clinically, this information is very important; but as an experiment to test the effects of vestibular stimulation, this provides unclear results.

Obviously no convenient solution exists to the problem of developing control groups in the clinic. Sometimes investigators must rely on statistical procedures or create a design where intervention effects are obvious. One example is to use a design similar to that used in some single subject research. For example a group of subjects is withheld from therapy long enough for a baseline to be obtained, intervention is introduced and then removed for the determination of another baseline. Withholding therapy could be brief and justified in order to make necessary assessments, and the group of subjects could serve as its own control group. A problem with this is that, if the intervention has permanent or long-lasting effects, then subsequent baseline assessments will not be informative. The control effect of the baseline would be counteracted by long-term effects of therapy. Inexperienced researchers, who want to come up with innovative control groups, are encouraged to consult with other more experienced experimenters, who can offer guidance in the development of the most effective, ethical, and efficient research designs.

Gathering Data as a Part of Daily Routine

We feel that data ultimately can be collected as a routine part of a therapist's day, but this should not interfere with regular responsibilities. Certainly other therapists and the administration should be informed of the nature and scope of the research project. Some facilities have their own libraries, and others will periodically give release time for therapists to conduct bibliographic research and to keep up with current trends in their fields. Most therapists are pressed for time, but there are ways to cut corners. For example, most facilities require in-service education presentations. Developing in-service programs around a topic which will be subsequently developed for a research project is a way of overlapping interests. Similarly, therapists have to perform initial evaluations on clients and to assess progress. Each of these measures can supply important data for a research project. Another time-saver is to divide responsibilties, taking advantage of others' expertise as well as the assistance of volunteers and students. A well-designed study can be broken down into manageable parts and can be conducted one part at a time. Additionally, if a research project requires very specific subjects that are not available in groups, subjects can be tested one at a time while still using principles of random sampling. Carefully designed, well thought-out research projects do not have to be so time-consuming that they interrupt other professional responsibilities.

Reporting the Same Data and Repeatedly Using the Same Subject Pool

It is inappropriate to publish the same research findings in multiple sources. Repeatedly using the same data and subjecting it to traditional probability levels violates statistical laws of probability. Additionally, most journals publish what is considered "original" research, and many journals require a statement that the work has not been published elsewhere. If the findings of a study have been presented first at a conference or as part of a Master's thesis, then this should be noted in a footnote to the journal article.

One of the frustrations of research, especially clinical research where it is difficult to establish controls, is that it is subject to confounding by extraneous variables. Caution should be exercised by researchers who make conclusions regarding data that have all been taken from the same subject pool. Sometimes research findings are a result of an exceptional (or deviant) subject pool, and the findings do not generalize to larger populations. At the least, researchers' conclusions should be tentative, and they should report the restrictions of their conclusions. An example of this appears in one of the studies discussed in this section: "Nystagmus and Ocular Fixation Difficulties in Learning-Disabled Children" (Reprint 5). In this study, we point out the procedural and theoretical limitations to the data. One of the limitations was the use of relatively few subjects, many of whom, "belonged to a group of children that has been extensively studied. Thus, the problem of sample-specific characteristics is particularly important with regard to this and to other related . . . projects." (Reprint 5, p. 721) Future research should clarify if our findings were sample-specific or whether they can be generalized.

General Guidelines

Ethical guidelines exist for conducting and publishing research. These are developed for particular institutions as well as for journals. To answer questions regarding publication ethics, author guides for specific journals can be consulted. New writers should be aware that different journals have different criteria and styles, and these should be consulted prior to writing and submitting a paper to any specific journal. In addition, journal editors or other experienced researchers can often offer suggestions and advice. Many professors and clinical researchers are excited about and willing to discuss their own research as well as give advice to others who are inexperienced but motivated to listen and learn. Published research and unpublished theses or dissertations, often available in college libraries, provide examples of procedures related to subject recruitment and selection, subject participation and authorization forms, and photographic release forms. One of the best ways to learn about actually doing research is to read research.

REFERENCES

1. Ayres AJ: *Sensory Integration and Learning Disorders*. Los Angeles, Western Psychological Services, 1972.

2. DeQuiros JB, Schrager OL: *Neuropsychological Fundamentals in Learning Disabilities*. San Rafael, CA, Academic Therapy Press, 1978.

Nystagmus and Ocular Fixation Difficulties in Learning-Disabled Children

Kenneth Ottenbacher
P. J. Watson
Margaret A. Short
Michael D. Biderman

ABSTRACT. The visual fixation ability of learning-disabled children was evaluated after sensory integrative therapy had been administered for short or long periods of time. Children with hyporesponsive postrotary nystagmus displayed reduced oculomotor control skills, but the deficit was apparent only in those who had been in therapy for a shorter interval. These results present further support for the hypothesis that the learning disabled can be differentiated according to their nystagmus characteristics. In addition, very tentative evidence suggested that sensory integrative therapy may have been successful in ameliorating the fixation deficiency; however, further research into this possibility is needed. The data also indicate that oculomotor control dysfunction may be a mediating mechanism for at least part of the learning disabilities experienced by some learning-disabled children.

Data obtained by a number of investigators suggest that learning-disabled (LD) children can be meaningfully categorized according to characteristics of their vestibular-proprioceptive systems. Ayres conducted a series of factor analytic studies in the early 1960s that revealed a subgroup of LD children characterized by poor postural responding, remnants of primitive postural reflexes, difficulty in coordinating the two sides of the body, and oculomotor incoordination.[1] Subsequent research has further supported the conclusion that some LD children exhibit a wide range of abnormal vestibular-proprioceptive traits.[2-6] In addition, during sensory integrative therapy, LD children with hyperactive postrotary nystagmus reactions have been found to display oculomotor[7] and academic[8] changes that are different from those of other LD children. Also, these children may display behavioral patterns that are different from those of other LD children;[9,10] however, the exact nature of the behavioral difference remains to be clearly delineated.[11]

This study examined further the subgroup of LD children with hyporesponsive nystagmus by assessing their visual fixation capabilities. It responded to the facts that the vestibular-proprioceptive system is intimately involved in controlling eye movements,[12] that eye movement control is important in such academic skills as reading,[13] and that visual fixation, saccadic, and visual pursuit movements are often abnormal in LD children.[14] Frank and Levinson[15] have already documented a relationship between dyslexia and dysfunction of the vestibular apparatus, cerebellum, and oculomotor system.

Ayres[8] recently reported that LD children with hyporeactive postrotary nystagmus responded to special education and sensory integrative therapy with greater improvements in reading and spelling than did LD children with average or above-average postrotary nystagmus durations. In contrast, LD children with subnormal nystagmus durations who received special education without sensory integrative therapy actually exhibited less improvement than the other LD groups. These findings suggest that LD children with hyporeactive nystagmus are sensitive to sensory integrative therapy in areas demanding eye movement control.

This study explored a possible explanation of these findings. DeQuiros and Schrager[9] claimed that hyporesponsive nystagmus is one symptom of a vestibular-oculomotor disturbance that results in an inability to efficiently maintain the eye movements necessary for reading. It had previously been demonstrated that sensory integrative therapy lengthens the postrotary nystagmus duration in some LD children with an initially low duration,[7] and this effect presumably rests on the use of activities that stimulate the vestibular system and thus takes advantage of the plasticity of this developing system. If a link exists between hyporesponsive nystagmus and the occurrence of oculomotor control dysfunction, then oculomotor deficiencies in these children should be reduced or eliminated as the postrotary nystagmus duration approaches normal levels. This hypothesis was examined by testing the prediction that LD children with initial hyporesponsive nystagmus would have deficient oculomotor control skills early in therapy before the full effect of vestibular stimulation could be achieved, while children further along in therapy would not display such a deficiency.

METHOD

Subjects included 27 male and 8 female children between 74 and 120 months of age. Data from many of them have been previously reported in regard to other issues.[5,7,10] All children had medical and/or educational diagnoses of learning disabilities or minimal brain dysfunction and had been referred by physicians to a children's rehabilitation center for diagnostic evaluation. Each child was individually administered the Southern California Sensory Integration Test (SCSIT) and the Southern California

Postrotary Nystagmus Test (SCPNT). Subjects were placed in sensory integrative therapy based on SCSIT and SCPNT results indicative of sensory integrative dysfunction. These judgments were made by two therapists experienced in pediatrics, one of whom was certified in the administration and interpretation of the SCSIT.

No distinct cut-off score was employed in assigning subjects to treatment; instead, clusters of scores were analyzed based on existing knowledge of sensory integrative dysfunction and previously identified syndromes.[16] Sensory integrative therapy consisted of planned activities designed to enhance the function and integration of the vestibular, proprioceptive, and tactile systems. Treatment was administered to small groups ranging from 2 to 5 children an average of 2 treatment hours per week. The emphasis during therapy was on vestibular-proprioceptive activities. These activities stressed passive and active rotary and linear movements and included various rolling games, the use of sit and spins, suspended net hammocks, inner tubes, and bolsters. A variety of scooterboard activities using a ramp were also employed. The children were generally allowed to alternately choose among the activities until all the children participated in all the activities. The length of time spent in therapy for individual subjects ranged from 1 to 29 months at the termination of the study.

The Saccadic Fixation Test, as described in the Pre Con Optometric training manual,[17] was used at the end of the study to measure ocular fixation ability. This test presented subjects with a sheet of paper on which a block of equally spaced letters was printed, 10 letters wide and 10 letters long. The subject was asked to read the first and last letter on each of the 10 lines, and both the time required for task completion and the number of errors were recorded. A final test score was obtained by multiplying task time in seconds by the ratio of 20 over 20 minus the number of errors. With such a procedure, lower scores indicated better performance.

All children were placed into one of four groups based on two factors, their original SCPNT scores and their length of time in sensory integrative therapy. Children with original SCPNT scores less than or equal to -1.0 were placed in a Low Nystagmus Group (LO), whereas all others were placed in a Comparison Nystagmus Group (COM). Within each nystagmus condition, the median duration of therapy was ascertained; and subjects below this median were assigned to a Short Therapy Group (Short), whereas all others were put in a Long Therapy Group (Long). In summary, the four groups were LO-Short, LO-Long, COM-Short, COM-Long. What the sex factor contributed to variability in ocular fixation scores was not formally analyzed because so few females were available for analysis and because Ayres[8] reported no sex-specific sensitivity to therapy. In addition, the nystagmus duration and ocular fixation scores of the LD girls were generally observed to be within the ranges of those of the LD boys. The SCPNT was periodically readministered throughout the study.

RESULTS

The characteristics of the groups are reviewed in Table 1, which reveals two points made previously.[7] First, LO subjects responded to sensory integrative therapy with reliable postrotary nystagmus duration increases $[t(18) = -2.53, p < .05]$, whereas other LD children displayed decreases $[t(15) = 5.46, p < .05]$. Second, these effects tended to be somewhat more apparent after relatively long treatment intervals. These

Table 1
Characteristics of Low and Comparison Nystagmus Group
after Relatively Short or Long Durations of Sensory Integrative Therapy

Characteristic	Low Nystagmus Group (Therapy)		Comparison Nystagmus Group (Therapy)	
	Short	Long	Short	Long
Children (N)				
Boys	7	10	6	4
Girls	2	0	2	4
Total	9	10	8	8
Age (Months)				
Boys $\bar{X}$	86.7	90.2	98.0	89.3
Range	76-98	81-110	74-120	85-99
Girls $\bar{X}$	86.0	—	87.0	97.8
Range	78-94	—	76-98	85-111
Total $\bar{X}$	86.6	90.2	95.3	93.5
Range	76-98	81-110	74-120	85-111
$\bar{X}$ Duration of Therapy (months)	4.4	10.7	5.0	17.3
$\bar{X}$ Initial Nystagmus Duration (sec)*	7.1	6.2	19.9	25.6
$\bar{X}$ Final Nystagmus Duration (sec)†	8.4	9.9	10.9	11.5
$\bar{X}$ Trend Score‡	.57	.64	.34	.32

*Duration of nystagmus during initial evaluation.
†Duration of nystagmus at end of study.
‡Trend Score = final nystagmus duration/initial plus final durations.

results were demonstrated in the mean initial and final nystagmus durations and in the mean trend scores (final nystagmus duration divided by
the sum of the initial and final durations).

The age data did present some interpretative difficulties because COM
subjects were somewhat older. Further, a correlative analysis indicated
that age tended to be correlated with therapy duration ($r = .23$ for LO
and $r = .15$ for COM children) and also with fixation score ($r = -.41$
for LO and $r = -.30$ for COM). This presented two problems. First, any
effects of therapy duration could be confounded with age because children who had been in therapy for relatively longer periods also tended to
be older. Second, the negative age-fixation correlations indicated that
older children scored better on the Saccadic Fixation Test. This meant
that the COM groups could exhibit significantly better fixation scores
because of age rather than because of variables related to nystagmus. An
analysis of covariance was used as a control for these problems. The use
of age as a covariate presented a statistical technique for sorting out the
influence of this variable, thus enabling an evaluation of the nystagmus
grouping and therapy duration effects.

Scores made on the fixation test are presented in Table 2. As it indicates, both LO groups scored higher (i.e., performed more poorly) than
did the COM groups. In addition, task performance within each condition
was poorer for those children who had received relatively less therapy;
but the difference was much more evident in the LO condition. The analysis of covariance verified statistically significant findings for the nystagmus grouping effect [$F(1, 30), = 5.31, p < .05$], for the therapy duration
effect [$F(1, 30) = 8.86, p < .05$], and for the nystagmus-by-duration interaction [$F(1,30) = 4.21, p < .05$]. The nature of these significant effects was examined in greater detail by employing t-tests, and it was
found that the LO group performed more poorly than the Comparison
group after short [$t(17) = 3.01, p < .01$] but not after long [$t(14) =
0.67, p < .05$] therapy duration. This pattern is consistent with the
prediction that LO LD children have deficient oculomotor control skills
before but not after therapy-related stimulation processes have had an opportunity to produce their full effect. The effect of the age covariate also
was statistically significant [$F(1, 30) = 8.20, p < .05$], but it should be
reemphasized that the nystagmus grouping and therapy effects cannot be
attributed to the age variable because the covariate analysis mathematical-
ly controlled for its influence.

Correlations also were used to analyze these fixation data. For the LO
groups, fixation scores were significantly related to trend scores ($r =
-.48, p < .05$) and to therapy duration ($r = -.69, p < .05$). In contrast,
neither of these correlations even approached significance ($r = -.10$,
both $p > .30$) for the COM subjects. Although possible influences of age
must be kept in mind, these correlations suggest that the use of the

Table 2
Saccadic Fixation Test Scores of Low and Comparison Groups
after Relatively Short or Long Durations of Sensory Integrative Therapy

		Therapy Duration Short	Long
Group			
Low Nystagmus	X̄	33.00*	18.90
	S D	13.14	6.57
Comparison Nystagmus	X̄	18.50	16.88
	S D	4.93	4.82

*Higher scores indicate poorer performance.

nystagmus and therapy duration variables in predicting fixation abilities may be particularly important in the subgroup of LD children with subnormal postrotary nystagmus durations.

DISCUSSION

De Quiros and Schrager[9] recently divided learning disability into a number of subcategories, one of which was labeled vestibular-oculomotor split. They stated, "When vestibular-oculomotor pathways functionally fail, fixation and skilled movements of the eyes (like those used to follow sequenced patterns, which are essential for reading) are seldom produced; and reading abilities are consequently disrupted." (p 106) Results of this investigation are consistent with such a conclusion, since LD children with abnormally low postrotary nystagmus durations were deficient in a task measuring oculomotor fixation when tested after a relatively short interval of sensory integrative therapy. In contrast, LO nystagmus children did not display a significant deficit at the end of a relatively long therapy interval; and this result presents the possibility that therapy may ameliorate the difficulty, presumably through the increased vestibular stimulation afforded by the treatment.

It is important to realize the procedural and theoretical limitations of these data. In regard to procedural factors, it should be emphasized that relatively few subjects were used, and many of them belonged to a group of children that has been extensively studied. Thus, the problem of sample-specific characteristics is particularly important with regard to this and to other related[5,7,10] projects. Another procedural consideration of importance is that a stronger argument for the effects of therapy on fixation ability could be made with subjects who are given the fixation test at initial evaluation and throughout treatment. This would enable a direct documentation of changes in fixation abilities as a function of therapy and of therapy-related nystagmus duration changes; therefore, an extension of this study is needed.

In terms of theoretical limitations, what these results do not say should be stressed. Because of the correlational nature of the evidence, the data do not prove that the physiological deficits revealed by subnormal post-rotary nystagmus cause an oculomotor deficiency, nor do they prove that sensory integrative therapy helps eliminate the problem. Certainly, however, logical arguments for these conclusions could be drawn from previous research and speculations.[e.g., 3,8,9] Finally, it would be unfair to conclude from these data that the learning disability of these children rested solely upon vestibular-oculomotor dysfunction and an associated disadvantage in academic tasks necessitating normal eye movement control. The possibility exists that such a deficit is at least part of the problem, but it would be unwarranted to conclude that it is the only problem.

These data do indicate that attention to the postrotary nystagmus of LD children can be used to delineate differences within the diagnosis. They further suggest that therapists should routinely use a direct measure of fixation abilities in their evaluations of LD children. Such a procedure could be important because it might aid therapists in their attempts to present children with optimal therapeutic opportunities, and because it might help uncover the mechanisms underlying certain types of learning disability.

REFERENCES

1. Ayres AJ: *The Development of Sensory Integrative Theory and Practice*, Dubuque, IA: Kendall/Hunt Publishing Co., 1974

2. Ayres AJ: Deficits in sensory integration in educationally handicapped children. *J Learn Disabil* 2: 160-168, 1969

3. Ayres AJ: *Sensory Integration and Learning Disorders*, Los Angeles: Western Psychological Services, 1972

4. DeQuiros, JB: Diagnosis of vestibular disorders in the learning disabled. *J Learn Disabil* 9: 50-58, 1976

5. Ottenbacher K: Identifying vestibular processing dysfunction in learning-disabled children. *Am J Occup Ther* 32: 217-221, 1978

6. Steinberg M, Rendle-Short J: Vestibular dysfunction in young children with minor neurological impairment. *Dev Med Child Neurol* 19: 639-651, 1977

7. Ottenbacher K, Short MA, Watson PJ: Nystagmus duration changes of learning-disabled children during sensory integrative therapy. *Percept Mot Skills* 48: 1159-1164, 1979

8. Ayres AJ: Learning disabilities and the vestibular system. *J Learn Disabil* 11: 30-41, 1978

9. De Quiros JB, Schrager O: *Neuropsychological Fundamentals in Learning Disabilities*, San Rafael, CA: Academic Therapy, 1978

10. Ottenbacher K, Watson PJ, Short MA: Association between nystagmus hyporesponsivity and behavioral problems in learning-disabled children. *Am J Occup Ther* 33: 317-322, 1979

11. Jung-Finocchiaro AC: Behavior characteristics in learning-disabled children with postural reflex dysfunction. *Am J Occup Ther* 28: 18-22, 1974

12. Melville-Jones G: The vestibular system for eye movement control. In *Eye Movements and*

Psychological Processes, RA Monty, JW Senders, Editors. Hillsdale, NJ: Lawrence Erlbaum Associates, 1976

13. Taylor EA: Ocular-motor processes and the act of reading. In *Basic Visual Processes and Learning Disability*, G Leisman, Editor. Springfield, IL: Charles C Thomas, 1976

14. Allen MJ: The role of vision in learning disorders. *J Learn Disabil* 10: 22-26, 1977

15. Frank J, Levinson HN: Dysmetric dyslexia and dyspraxia. *Acad Ther* 11: 133-143, 1975-76

16. Ayres AJ: *Interpreting the Southern California Sensory Integration Tests*, Los Angeles: Western Psychological Services, 1976

17. Vincentt WK: *Optometric and Perception Testing and Training Manual*, Akron, OH: Pre Con Inc., 1975

Association Between Nystagmus Hyporesponsivity and Behavioral Problems in Learning-Disabled Children

Kenneth Ottenbacher
P. J. Watson
Margaret A. Short

ABSTRACT. This study explored the hypothesis that an association exists between postrotary nystagmus hyporesponsivity and behavioral problems in learning-disabled children. Supporting this conclusion was the finding that the learning-disabled boys rated by teachers as displaying the most socially inappropriate behaviors had significantly lower postrotary nystagmus durations than other learning-disabled boys. In addition, near significant associations were obtained between subnormal nystagmus functioning and socially inappropriate responding for boys and girls combined. Learning-disabled girls were evaluated as responding significantly more appropriately than learning-disabled boys, while having significantly shorter postrotary nystagmus durations; thus, sex of a child may be an important variable in determining relationships between psychological characteristics and hyporesponsive nystagmus. Additional research is needed in this area because of a number of limitations to this study; however, these results present further suggestive evidence that learning-disabled children can be categorized according to characteristics of their postrotary nystagmus.

Vestibular processing dysfunctions have been identified in a sizeable proportion of learning-disabled (LD) children, with symptoms including muscle hypotonicity, hyporeactive postrotary nystagmus, and poorly integrated postural reflexes and reactions.[1-6] The demonstration of these dysfunctions within the LD diagnosis has led to suggestions that clinically significant subgroups of learning disability can be delineated. The hypothesis has been presented that the learning disabilities of some children are caused by vestibular dysfunction and that treatment of the educational difficulty should include activities to improve the processing of vestibular and proprioceptive information.[2,3,6] Treatment principles and suggested therapeutic approaches have been developed by Ayres.[1,7] The activities, when properly applied, appear to ameliorate some forms of learning disability, particularly those characterized by hyporesponsive postrotary nystagmus. Further research designed to explore the vestibular characteristics of these children therefore has implications for professionals working in this area.

One way in which LD children with deficits in vestibular abilities may differ from other LD children is in their behavioral characteristics. DeQuiros and Schrager recently argued that vestibular processing impairments often lead to learning disabilities and that symptoms associated with these conditions include "restlessness," "distractibility," and a "super-imposed emotional disturbance."[6] Linkages between vestibular dysfunction and behavioral abnormalities have been suggested by studies where children referred to a child guidance clinic were examined,[9] and where children were diagnosed as hyperactive,[10] dyslexic,[11] emotionally disturbed,[12] and autistic.[13]

The purpose of this study was to determine whether or not an association exists between nystagmus hyporesponsivity and behavior problems in LD children. Based on the DeQuiros and Schrager[6] hypothesis, and on the results of previous research,[e.g., 10,12,13] it was hypothesized that LD children with behavioral problems would display greater evidence of hyporeactive postrotary nystagmus. This general issue was investigated previously by Jung-Finocchiaro who examined two groups of LD boys, one of which evidenced deficits on three measures of postural reflex function.[14] She found a significant relationship between degree of postural dysfunction and external reliance, a factor on the Devereux Elementary School Behavior Rating Scale that measures passivity.[15] However, the significance level used in this study was .10; and, since the Devereux scale has 11 factors, one significant result would be expected by chance. It should be noted that Jung-Finocchiaro also found near significant relationships on two other factors, indicating that the boys with postural problems tended to be more inattentive and withdrawn and to have less well-developed interactions with the teacher. In addition, a higher incidence of conduct disorders, as measured by the Devereux Scale, was reported in the LD boys without postural reflex abnormalities.[14] This result suggested that LD boys without vestibular abnormalities were more likely to display rowdiness, disruptiveness, fighting, irresponsibility, destructiveness, irritability, and dislike for school.[14] This outcome is counter to that predicted from the DeQuiros and Schrager hypothesis. Jung-Finocchiaro argued that the behavioral pattern of the children without postural reflex dysfunction was consistent with "the expected developmental pattern of boys' behavior" and that the obtained results served as further indication of a developmental lag experienced by LD children with postural reflex dysfunction.[14] Nevertheless, it is apparent that the behavioral attributes of LD children with evidence of impaired vestibular capabilities have not been clearly delineated, and that additional research is needed in this area.

METHOD

Thirty-one boys and 14 girls between the ages of 51 and 114 months participated in this investigation. All subjects had either a medical or an educational diagnosis (or both) of learning disability and had been referred by physicians to a children's rehabilitation center for diagnostic testing and treatment. Intelligence quotients were within normal range, 80-120, as far as could be determined from psychological and school reports. Diagnostic testing included the administration of the Southern California Postrotary Nystagmus Test (SCPNT),[16] which provides a direct measure of vestibular-ocular reflexes (postrotary nystagmus) in children five to ten years of age. The results of this test were employed for data analysis. Tests for all children were individually administered in a well-lighted room per standardized instructions by two therapists experienced in pediatrics.

As a part of the diagnostic work-up, teachers were asked to rate each child on a behavioral rating scale designed by rehabilitation center personnel. The scale included 21 items thought to characterize children with behavior disorders. Individual items were scored on a 3-point scale with: 1—behavior never observed; 2—behavior occasionally observed; and 3—behavior usually observed. The items presented on the scale are listed in Table 1.

For purposes of data analysis, nystagmus durations obtained on the SCPNT were compared with normative data to determine group assignment. All subjects with SCPNT scores of more than 1 standard deviation below the mean were placed in the hyporesponsive or Low Nystagmus Group. The remaining children made up the Control Group.

RESULTS

Median scores on the behavioral rating scale were computed for each child, and examination of these data revealed obvious differences between the boys and the girls. Eleven out of the 31 males received a median rating of 3, whereas no females received such a score; this difference was statistically significant (Fisher's exact test, $p < .01$, two-tailed test).

This sex difference complicated the statistical examination of the data. First, the ratings of the boys were analyzed by assigning Low Nystagmus and Control subjects to a Socially Appropriate (SA) or Socially Inappropriate (SI) behavior group. Determination of behavior group placement was made by assigning males with the highest median behavioral ratings (median > 2.0) to the SI group and the remaining males to the SA group. Using this procedure, 6 of 11 Low Nystagmus subjects fell in the SI category, whereas only 5 of 20 Controls did so, a result that approached sta-

Table 1

Items on Behavior Rating Scale

---

1. Disruptiveness, frequently annoys or bothers others
2. Restlessness, inability to sit still
3. Short attention span
4. Fighting
5. Temper tantrum
6. Tension, inability to relax
7. Has difficulty communicating, speech is hard to understand
8. Disobedience, difficulty in disciplinary control
9. Uncooperative in group situations
10. Hyperactive, always on the go
11. Distractableness
12. Destructiveness in regard to own or other's property or both
13. Profane language
14. Nervousness, jitteriness, jumpiness, easily startled
15. Irritability, hot tempered, easily aroused to anger
16. Excessive talking
17. Requires adult supervision or attendance constantly
18. Inability for quiet play
19. Constantly changes activities
20. Disrupts other's play
21. Interrupts teacher and other children

tistical significance (Fisher's test, $p = .11$, one-tailed test). Since no female obtained a median rating greater than 2.0, placement of girls into the SI category occurred with a median equal to 2.0. Five of the ten Low Nystagmus females, but only one of four Controls, were categorized in the SI group. Although such a pattern of results is consistent with the hypothesis that girls with hyporeactive postrotary nystagmus are also more likely to display relatively less appropriate behaviors, the small number of female subjects prevented this outcome from approaching statistical significance (Fisher's test, $p > .20$, one-tailed test). Finally, a composite 2×2 matrix was composed by collapsing across the sex variable and adding Low Nystagmus-SI males and females together, and so on for the other three cells. Such an approach produced a matrix in which Low Nystagmus and Control children were categorized as displaying SI behavior if their responses were poor *relative* to other same-sexed subjects. In this instance, 11 of 21 Low Nystagmus children were placed in the SI behavior group, whereas only 6 of 24 controls were similarly assigned, a result that again approached statistical significance (Fisher's test, $p = .06$, one-tailed test).

The strongest evidence of a tie between nystagmus hyporesponsivity and behavioral functioning was obtained when the nystagmus durations of males in the SI and SA groups were compared. SI males had a mean nystagmus duration of 14.73 sec (SD = 6.66), and the mean for the SA males was 21.95 sec (SD = 11.52). This difference was statistically significant [$t(29) = 1.90, p < .05$, one-tailed test]. The SA (M = 8.63 sec, SD = 7.71) and SI (M = 9.17 sec, SD = 6.18) females had nystagmus durations that were essentially the same [$t(12) = 0.14, p > .20$, one-tailed test].

An item-by-item analysis of the behavioral ratings was also conducted. For the males, no significant relationship between behavioral grouping and hyporesponsive nystagmus was obtained for any item; however, data from five items approached significance. As Table 2 reveals, the pattern of results from each near-significant outcome indicated that the percentage of SI boys within each nystagmus condition was higher for the Low Nystagmus subjects than for the Controls, and, in fact, this basic pattern was observed for 18 of the 21 behavioral characteristics. For the females, only two behavioral ratings approached significance (see Table 2). Both findings were also consistent with the hypothesis of an association between hyporeactive nystagmus and behavioral problems; however, it should be noted that this number of near-significant results could have occurred by chance. Overall, a pattern of results consistent with the hypothesis was obtained for only 12 of 21 behavioral ratings for females.

Table 2
Near-Significant Associations between Number* of Boys and Girls in Each Nystagmus and Behavior Group

Behavioral Characteristic	Low Nystagmus		Control		
	SA†	SI†	SA	SI	p‡
Males:					
1. Fighting	7	3	18	1	.07
2. Disobedience	6	5	17	3	.08
3. Hyperactive	3	8	12	8	.08
4. Disruptiveness	3	8	11	8	.11
5. Destructiveness	8	3	18	1	.13
Females:					
1. Communication Difficulty	4	6	4	0	.07
2. Disobedience	8	2	4	0	.13

• The number of children listed for each behavioral characteristic differs because teachers occasionally failed to respond to each item for each child.
† SA = Socially Appropriate; SI = Socially Inappropriate.
‡ Probability values were obtained by using one-tailed Fisher's tests.

The ages of the children were also analyzed. Low Nystagmus males (M = 79.56 months, SD = 7.80) were younger than the Control males (M = 87.15 months, SD = 17.28), but this difference failed to reach significance [$t(29) = 1.38, p > .10$, two-tailed test]. For females, Low Nystagmus subjects (M = 78.7 months, SD = 10.34) also were younger than controls (M = 87.25 months, SD = 22.02), but not significantly so [$t(12) = .93, p > .10$, two-tailed test]. With the males and females combined, the younger age of Low Nystagmus children (M = 79.14 months, SD = 8.57) was close to being significantly different [$t(43) = 1.43, p > .05$, two-tailed test] from the mean Control age of 87.17 months (SD = 17.61). Thus, the age data present some interpretative difficulties because children more likely to display socially inappropriate behaviors also exhibited a strong, although nonsignificant, tendency to be younger. However, when the ages were analyzed in terms of the SI versus SA Behavior Groups, none of the effects even approached significance. This was true of the boys [SI M = 81.18 months, SA M = 86.3 months, $t(29) = .91$, $p > .10$], of the girls [SI M = 82.33 months, SA M = 80.13 months, $t(12) = .26, p > .10$].

One final analysis revealed that the male subjects as a whole had significantly longer nystagmus durations (M = 19.42, SD = 10.55) than the females (M = 8.86 sec, SD = 5.84) with $t(43) = 3.42, p < .01$, two-tailed test. This result agrees with Ayres' standardization data for the SCPNT, which revealed significant differences in postrotary nystagmus durations based on sex. In the context of this investigation, such a finding suggests that hyporesponsive nystagmus as measured by the SCPNT may not be a sufficient condition for predicting the display of maladaptive behaviors. The reason for this is that the girls had significantly shorter nystagmus durations, yet were rated as displaying significantly more appropriate responses.

DISCUSSION

This investigation tested the hypothesis that LD children with more numerous behavioral problems present greater evidence of nystagmus hyporesponsivity. Support for this conclusion was obtained with the findings that a near-significant association existed between low nystagmus and socially inappropriate behavior in boys; that LD boys and girls taken together tended to exhibit a linkage between behavioral problems and hyporesponsive postrotary nystagmus; that SI boys had significantly lower nystagmus durations than SA boys; and that 18 out of 21 items on the boys' behavioral rating scales yielded a pattern consistent with the hypothesis. In addition, it was found that the behavior of LD boys was rated by teachers to be significantly poorer than that of LD girls and that LD girls had a significantly shorter nystagmus duration than LD boys.

Data obtained for LD females presented no substantive indication of an association between subnormal vestibular-oculomotor activity and behavioral problems. It was true that the percentage of girls in the SI group was higher for Low Nystagmus subjects than for Controls, and that 12 out of 21 items on the girls' rating scales produced a pattern congruent with the hypothesis; but it was also true that SA girls had a nonsignificantly lower average nystagmus duration than did SI girls. Thus, some very weak evidence was found both for and against the hypothesized relationship. Two reasons suggest caution in using these data to reach conclusions about the behavior of LD girls. First, only a relatively small number of females was available for analysis; and second, only a small number of these served as controls. Further experimental examination of LD females is therefore especially needed.

Overall, the results of this study produced some support for the hypothesis of DeQuiros and Schrager[6] that LD children with vestibular processing difficulties experience a "superimposed emotional disturbance." However, this investigation suggested that the behavioral difficulties may be largely a male phenomenon, although the limitations of the female data again must be kept in mind. The obtained sex difference in behavior may be a simple extension of normally observed patterns[17] and may be a reflection of social role expectations, but the fact that LD boys were rated overall as displaying significantly greater behavioral problems while having significantly longer nystagmus durations further strengthens the notion that the sex of a child is an important variable in determining possible associations between postrotary nystagmus and psychological characteristics.

Another important aspect of these results is that they differ from those reported by Jung-Finocchiaro. She observed that LD males with vestibular processing dysfunction as measured by postural reflex difficulties tended to withdraw from the environment and to be more passive than other LD boys, but the Low Nystagmus LD boys here seemed to exhibit more active, aggressive response modes. Procedural differences could explain this discrepancy because Jung-Finocchiaro used different criteria in identifying vestibular dysfunction; thus she may have explored different physiological systems. In fact, DeQuiros and Schrager have isolated two different learning disabilities related to vestibular dysfunction, vestibular-proprioceptive dissociation and vestibular-oculomotor split. Jung-Finocchiaro may have examined children more appropriately placed in the vestibular-proprioceptive dissociation group, whereas this study examined children in the vestibular-oculomotor split group.

In addition, Jung-Finocchiaro employed different psychological instruments, and this may have helped yield a different pattern of results. A final possibility also may deserve consideration. Assuming, as Ayres does,[2] that a causal relationship exists between sensory integration disorders and lowered adaptive skill, LD children with vestibular processing deficits may be limited in their ability to make appropriate responses to their environment. The way these children behaviorally manifest their lowered skill in turn may be determined by the environment. In some situations, they may withdraw, while in others they may become aggressive. Such an argument is speculative; and it is presented not so much as an explanation but as a plausible alternative that deserves experimental consideration.

The age data are somewhat problematic, since children with hyporesponsive nystagmus tended to be younger. Thus, the possibility exists that the behavioral correlates of the LD subgroups could have been linked to age rather than postrotary nystagmus differences. In other words, Low Nystagmus SI boys could have displayed more socially inappropriate responses simply because they were more immature. Two points argue against such an interpretation. First, the observed age differences were not statistically significant; but more importantly, the age data organized in terms of the SA versus the SI Groups did not yield results even approaching significance. This latter finding is particularly counter to any age-related explanation. A possible reason why Low Nystagmus children tended to be younger could be that they may present more discriminable evidence of their difficulties; and therefore, professionals may be able to identify them sooner.

By no means are the findings of this study presented as the definitive statement about the behavioral characteristics of LD children with hyporesponsive nystagmus. These data cannot be employed to draw firm conclusions because of the small number of females that served as subjects, the age differences in the group, the use of a nonstandardized behavioral instrument, and the conflicting results presented by Jung-Finocchiaro. Further, even the most clear-cut outcomes from this type of research design cannot be used to infer causality between variables. In other words, it is not possible to claim that vestibular-oculomotor deficits as measured by hyporesponsive postrotary nystagmus cause behavioral problems.

IMPLICATIONS FOR OCCUPATIONAL THERAPY

Nevertheless, the data are suggestive and have at least two implications for occupational therapists. First, they suggest that therapists may be able to use the behavioral characteristics of LD boys as one source of information employed in the diagnostic process. Postrotary nystagmus hyporesponsivity can be influenced by such variables as environmental lighting,[18] arousal level, and visual fixation;[19] and these factors can produce results that could be interpreted incorrectly as evidence of a physiological abnormality. Therefore, supplementary behavioral information may eventually prove helpful in strengthening the therapist's confidence in the evaluation of LD boys.

Second, and perhaps more importantly, data such as these serve as further support for the argument made by occupational therapists that postrotary nystagmus is a variable of therapeutic interest. DeQuiros and Schrager[6] have pointed out that the medical profession has tended to reject the rotary test of nystagmus as useful "because excitations elicited by it pertain not only to vestibular but also to many central structures."[6, p156] Therefore, the current use of this measure by occupational therapists stands in some contrast to the medical position. Although it is true that postrotary nystagmus may not be useful in defining the functional properties of specific physiological systems, it still may be a valid index of other processes. For example, Ayres[8] recently demonstrated the predictive validity of this measure by showing that the presence of postrotary nystagmus hyporeactivity can be used to reveal which LD children will be most responsive to sensory integrative therapy. The association between nystagmus hyporesponsivity and behavioral problems in LD boys uncovered in this study helps supply concurrent validity for the measure; and to the extent that these findings can be replicated, the claim will be strengthened for the existence of clinically significant subgroups of LD children categorized according to their postrotary nystagmus characteristics.

REFERENCES

1. Ayres, AJ: Deficits in sensory integration in educationally handicapped children. *J Learn Disabil* 2: 160-168, 1969

2. Ayres AJ: *Sensory Integration and Learning Disroders*, Los Angeles: Western Psychological Services, 1972

3. DeQuiros, JB: Diagnosis of vestibular disorders in the learning disabled. *J Learn Disabil* 9: 50-58, 1976

4. Ottenbacher K: Identifying vestibular processing dysfunction in learning-disabled children. *Am J Occup Ther* 32: 217-221, 1978

5. Steinberg M, Rendle-Short J: Vestibular dysfunction in young children with minor neurological impairment. *Dev Med Child Neurol* 19: 639-651, 1977

6. DeQuiros JB, Schrager O: *Neuropsychological Fundamentals in Learning Disabilities*, San Rafael, CA: Academic Therapy, 1978

7. Ayres AJ: Improving academic scores through sensory integration. *J Learn Disabil* 5: 338-343, 1972

8. Ayres, AJ: Learning disabilities and the vestibular system. *J Learn Disabil* 11: 30-41, 1978

9. Silberzahn M: Sensory integrative function in a child guidance clinic population. *Am J Occup Ther* 29: 86-91, 1975

10. Bhatara V, Clark DL, Arnold LE: Behavioral and nystagmus response of a hyperkinetic child to vestibular stimulation. *Am J Occup Ther* 32: 311-316, 1978

11. Frank J, Levinson HN: Dysmetric dyslexia and dyspraxia. *Acad Ther* 11: 133-143, 1975

12. Piggot L, Purcell O, Cummings G, Caldwell D: Vestibular dysfunction in emotionally disturbed children. *Biol Psychiatr* 11: 719-728, 1976

13. Ritvo EZ, Ornitz EM, Eviatar A, et al: Decreased postrotary nystagmus in early infantile autism. *Neurol* 19: 653-658, 1969

14. Jung-Finocchiaro AC: Behavior characteristics in learning-disabled children with postural relfex dysfunction. *Am J Occup Ther* 28: 18-22, 1974

15. Spivack G, Swift M: *Devereux Elementary School Behavior Rating Scale Manual*, Devon: The Devereux Foundation, 1967

16. Ayres AJ: *Southern California Postrotary Nystagmus Test*, Los Angeles: Western Psychological Services, 1975

17. Werry JS, Quay, HC: The prevalence of behavior symptoms in younger elementary school children. *Am J Orthopsychiatr* 41: 136-143, 1971

18. Levy D, Proctor L, Holzman P: Visual interference on vestibular response. *Arch Otolaryngol* 103: 287-291, 1977

19. Cogan D: *Neurology of the Ocular Muscles*, Second Edition. Springfield, IL: Charles C Thomas, 1956

PART 4:
A BODY OF COLLABORATIVE RESEARCH

The two articles included in Part 3 "Nystagmus and Ocular Fixation Difficulties in Learning Disabled Children" (Reprint 5) and "Association Between Nystagmus Hyporesponsivity and Behavioral Problems in Learning-Disabled Children" (Reprint 6) lend support to the conclusion that a specific type of learning disability can be differentiated according to measures of nystagmus duration. Additional hypotheses were made regarding this group of children. Some of these involved predicting how this group would respond to sensory integrative therapy, and a separate hypothesis was made in regard to these children's self-images. From examination of the intake evaluations, these children were not able to portray themselves adequately through a draw-a-person task, and existing research supported that observation.[1]

Additional support for this observation came from our previous finding regarding the reduced ocular fixation abilities of learning disabled children with hyporesponsive nystagmus. We hypothesized that poor ocular fixation would interfere with perception of self and with the ability to portray manually an accurate human body that consisted of proportional, sufficient body parts. In the study, "Human Figure Drawings of Learning Disabled Children with Hyporesponsive Postrotary Nystagmus" (Reprint 7), we assessed this ability and confirmed the original clinical observations that the children with low durations of nystagmus produced inferior human figure drawings when compared to a group of children with medium or high durations of nystagmus.

SINGLE SUBJECT RESEARCH

Ken's study, "Patterns of Postrotary Nystagmus in Three Learning Disabled Children" (Reprint 8) added to our understanding of nystagmus and learning disabilities. The advantages to this study are that Ken sampled from an entirely different subject pool which we had not previously examined in our line of research. Also, he used a different methodology than we had previously used. The single subject method which he selected can be very useful for therapists who have limited resources for testing and treating the large groups of subjects required for many experimental designs. The single subject design, if used properly, can be very informative, although it has drawbacks. For example, the illness of a subject or one subject's withdrawal from such a study can terminate the entire project. In addition, generalizations from a single subject study are limited, but the findings can be used to suggest directions for other investigations.

HOW TO DEAL WITH CONFOUNDING VARIABLES

The results of the study "Patterns of Postrotary Nystagmus in Three Learning Disabled Children" (Reprint 8) are consistent with the findings of our other studies and are in line with predictions made from clinical observations and from theory. Those predictions are that learning disabled children who exhibit hyporesponsive nystagmus will display nystagmus duration increases after exposure to treatment using sensory integration procedures. Children with normal ranges of nystagmus duration are expected, after repeated vestibular stimulation, to display habituation, resulting in diminished prn durations.[2,3] These predictions, however, posed some difficulties for us when it came time to interpret the results of our studies.

In statistical descriptions of behavior, a phenomenon termed regression toward the mean predicts that extremes of behavior, as a matter of course, tend to drift (or regress) toward normal. In our studies, low durations of nystagmus increased over time (and with therapy), while higher durations decreased. While this is exactly what we predicted, these findings could also be interpreted as artifactual—due to regression toward the mean. Thus, even though our studies confirmed clinical and theoretical predictions, the findings could be interpreted as statistically artifactual. Regression toward the mean would make the same prediction as theory and cannot be sorted out of these current studies. This is discussed specifically in regard to our predictions in the manuscript, "Nystagmus Duration Changes of Learning Disabled Children During Sensory Integrative Therapy" (Reprint 9).

Certainly a researcher's confidence is increased when experimental findings verify predictions based on clinical observations *and* are supported by theory. While confounding variables make conclusions tentative and necessitate cautions in interpreting results, several methods can be used to reduce their interference. One is to use statistical procedures to reduce or eliminate their contribution, and another is to conduct additional studies that are designed specifically to examine their effects. An additional way to put confounding variables into perspective is to examine them within a broader context.

Statistical Analysis

Because the variable, age, had posed possible problems in the two studies discussed in Part 3, we used an analysis that enabled us statistically to minimize the contribution of that factor. The Analysis of Covariance is a statistical procedure that enables the experimenter to compare certain variables while holding constant the effects of another, potentially confounding variable. In the study, "Human Figure Drawings of Learning Disabled Children With Hyporesponsive Postrotary Nystagmus" (Reprint 7), we used this procedure, treating age as a covariate, while investigating the effects of nystagmus duration on human figure drawing performance. Certainly the results of the study were consistent with our predictions, but other interpretations could also be made. One possible interpretation that an editorial reviewer pointed out to us is that the children with low nystagmus may have also possessed less intellectual ability. This would account for the inferior skills with human figure drawings, and *could* possibly be responsible for the findings of our other studies. Thus, the behavioral problem, ocular fixation difficulties, as well as the poorer human figure drawings could result, not from vestibular-related problems, as we had suggested, but to inferior intellectual abilities. This suggestion obviously was frustrating to us, as the studies had been published, and we were excited that our findings confirmed clinical expectations as well as theoretical predictions. We did not have access to I.Q. data based on individually administered tests for all of the children in that study, so we were unable to assess directly whether our groups differed on this variable.

Isolating and Addressing Confounding Variables

Ottenbacher, Abbot, Haley and Watson, however, addressed that problem with their study which is also reported here. The results of this investigation, "Human Figure Drawing Ability and Vestibular Processing Dysfunction in Learning Disabled Children" (Reprint 10), confirmed that human figure drawing scores and prn are related. In addition, IQ data were analyzed, and the results indicated that IQ was not significantly related to prn durations and, therefore, was not a confounding factor.

This study is an excellent example of an investigation that is systematically designed to clarify previous research and to sort out and identify variables. While this study addressed the confound introduced by the IQ variable, other carefully planned studies could also address the problem introduced by regression toward the mean. For example, regression toward the mean would be negated by carefully designed experimental studies illustrating changes in nystagmus durations of one treated group but not in a differently treated group of low prn learning disabled children. Matching those groups on IQ data would additionally eliminate the other potential confound. Nystagmus changes observed in the same subjects under one treatment condition but not in a different treatment would also address the regression problem.

INTERPRETING RESEARCH FROM A CONTEXT

The fact that any one study possesses a specific design or methodological weakness means that the results of that single study may be open to multiple interpretation. When the study is considered within the larger context of studies exploring the same or similar research hypotheses, however, the results can contribute to the validation of a theory or a treatment technique. Suppose, for example, that in a collection of 100 studies, studies #1-20 are weak in representative sampling but otherwise strong; studies #21-30 are weak in terms of internal validity; studies #31-40 are weak in relation to the type of data analysis used, and so on. But imagine that all 100 studies are similar in that they demonstrate a superiority of the treatment (intervention) over the control or comparison groups. The critic who maintains that the total collection of studies does *not* support the conclusion of treatment efficacy is forced to invoke an explanation of multiple causality (i.e., the reported effect can be caused by either this particular design flaw, or this particular analysis flaw, or this particular measurement flaw). The number of multiple causes which must be invoked to counter the explanation of treatment efficacy can be large even for a few dozen studies. Indeed, the multiple defects explanation soon develops into a conspiracy theory or else collapses under its own weight. The point is that it is important to place any given study within a context of a larger body of research literature.

SIGNIFICANCE OF OUR RESEARCH

Collectively, our studies addressed a very specific type of learning disability. The value of understanding the characteristics of this population is significant. One such value is the ability to predict whether a specific target population responds positively to therapy. This was one of our goals in the studies: "Nystagmus Duration Changes of Learning Disabled Children During Sensory Integrative Therapy" (Reprint 9), "The Use of Selected Clinical Observations to Predict Postrotary Nystagmus Change in Learning Disabled Children" (Reprint 11), and "Patterns of Postrotary Nystagmus in Three Learning Disabled Children" (Reprint 8). In Part 2, we noted that certain clinical variables were predictors of nystagmus. We then hypothesized that a certain population of learning disabled children existed who would be sensitive to sensory integrative therapy.

This specific population could be delineated by what we called "vestib-ular-proprioceptive" (V-P) characteristics. We speculated that the learn-ing disabled children with low prn durations, low muscle tone, and poor balance, would respond to therapy with increased durations of prn. Clin-ically, we felt from observation that this particular group of children was responding to therapy; and predictions from theory supported this obser-vation. Ayres[4] had claimed that the vestibular systems of children with low prn would "normalize" after exposure to sensory integrative pro-cedures. We interpreted normalization to mean that their nystagmus re-sponses would gradually increase to the standardized normal measures.[5]

All three studies confirmed our hypotheses regarding the prn responses of low nystagmus learning disabled children who are exposed to therapy using sensory integrative procedures. Furthermore, the results of the study, "The Use of Selected Clinical Observations to Predict Postrotary Nystagmus Change in Learning Disabled Children" (Reprint 11) indi-cated that we could predict which specific group of learning disabled chil-dren would respond. In this study, learning disabled children with low nystagmus were further separated based on additional vestibular-proprio-ceptive characteristics. Of the group that had other V-P deficits, 11 of 12 children responded to therapy with increases in the duration of nystag-mus. In our comparison group of children without deficits in balance and antigravity postures, only one-half responded with increases in nystagmus after therapy.

One conclusion that may be made from the findings of these studies is that learning disabled children with hyporesponsive prn actually improve during therapy, but this conclusion can only be tentative. Can we con-clusively claim that increases in nystagmus duration signify improve-ment? Were the children in therapy really getting better? On what skills were they demonstrating improvements? In retrospect, we should have added other components to our study. For example, we could have in-cluded some pre- and post-treatment measures of improvement other than prn. For example, did other V-P measures also change at the same time as prn did? Did muscle tone, balance, prone extension posture, ocular fix-ation, or drawing abilities improve?

One of Ayres' studies[6] supported the findings of these studies, as she reported that the academic scores of children with low prn increased after sensory integration therapy. Unfortunately we did not have measures of academic performance, and Ayres, in her study, did not report any pre-post differences in nystagmus. One piece of evidence that did support our findings is from the previously discussed study, "Nystagmus and Ocular Fixation Difficulties in Learning Disabled Children" (Reprint 5). In this study, we looked at children with short or long durations of nystagmus, and we also examined whether their ocular fixation scores differed de-pending upon the length of their participation in therapy. We found that ocular fixation was better in the low prn group that had been exposed to longer durations of therapy.

Collectively, all of our studies had consistencies. Our original clinical observations were validated, and the collection of studies, even with confounds and limitations, was exciting because new ideas were generated by every new study. Additionally, our other research[7,8] was contributing to a body of information regarding nystagmus and various clinical populations.

REFERENCES

1. DeQuiros JB, Schrager OL: *Neuropsychological Fundamentals in Learning Disabilities*. San Rafael, CA, Academic Therapy Press, 1978.

2. Crampton GH: Habituation of ocular nystagmus of vestibular origin, in Bender M (ed.): *The Oculomotor System*. New York, Harper & Row, 1964.

3. Johnson D, Torok N: Habituation of nystagmus and sensation of motion after rotation. *Acta Otolaryngol* 69:206-215, 1970.

4. Ayres AJ: *Sensory Integration and Learning Disorders*. Los Angeles, Western Psychological Services, 1972.

5. Ayres AJ, Heskett W: Sensory integrative dysfunction in a young schizophrenic girl. *J Aut Child Schizophrenia* 2:174-181, 1972.

6. Ayres AJ: Learning disabilities and the vestibular system. *J Learn Disabil* 11:30-41, 1978.

7. Ottenbacher K: Excessive postrotary nystagmus duration in learning-disabled children. *Am J Occup Ther* 34:40-44, 1980.

8. Watson PJ, Ottenbacher K, Workman EA, Short MA, Dickman DA: Visual motor difficulties in emotionally disturbed children with hyporesponsive nystagmus. *Phys Occup Ther Pediatr* 2(2/3):67-72, 1982.

Human Figure Drawings
of Learning Disabled Children with
Hyporesponsive Postrotary Nystagmus

P.J. Watson
Kenneth Ottenbacher
Margaret A. Short
Jane Kittrell
Edward A. Workman

ABSTRACT. The Southern California Postrotary Nystagmus Test (SCPNT) was administered to 52 children who were asked to sketch human figure drawings (HFD) during assessment procedures designed to determine learning disability and perceptual motor dysfunction. Analysis of these data confirmed the hypothesis that children with hyporesponsive nystagmus would display less skill in their HFD performance than those with longer postrotary nystagmus (PRN) durations. The suggestions that therapists should assess the vestibular characteristics of these children were supported by the results of this study; however, a definitive statement concerning PRN and HFD relationships must await additional research. Future investigations will need to ensure that the PRN-HFD associations are not mediated by one or more of the other variables found to be correlated with HFD performance.

Contemporary analyses of learning disabilities have included neuropsychological investigations into vestibular-proprioceptive variables. Ayres,[1] for example, has identified a subgroup of learning disabled (LD) children characterized by abnormal postrotary nystagmus (PRN), muscle hypotonicity, and poorly integrated postural reactions. She also has reported that LD children with hyporesponsive postrotary nystagmus are particularly sensitive to remediation efforts when attempts are made to redress their vestibular-proprioceptive deficits.[2] Other researchers have concurred that vestibular-proprioceptive functioning may be important in evaluating and treating these children.[3-7]

In this investigation, children assessed for learning disabilities and perceptual-motor dysfunction were asked to sketch human figure drawings (HFD)[8] and were administered the Southern California Postrotary Nystagmus Test (SCPNT).[9] Three lines of reasoning were used in hypothesizing that children with a hyporesponsive nystagmus would display poorer HFD performance than children exhibiting relatively longer PRN durations. First, DeQuiros and Schrager[3] have argued that a "superimposed emotional disturbance" often accompanies vestibular abnormalities; and global ratings of the HFD may be sensitive to "gross maladjustment".[8] Second, and more important, the existence of hyporesponsive postrotary nystagmus suggests suboptimal vestibular-oculomotor coordination; and such incoordination, when combined with hand movements, might result in a writing[3] or drawing disability. Swenson[8] has concluded that drawing ability is a significant source of variance in HFD performance, and children with reduced vestibular-oculomotor control skill consequently may be less able to draw. Third, Culp and associates[10] recently reported that the figure drawing performance of preschoolers was improved by a sensorimotor training program that included attention to vestibular input, and their observations further suggest a linkage between vestibular system functioning and ability to draw human figures.

METHOD

Subjects

Fifty-two children (31 males and 21 females) ranging in age from 66 to 136 months served as subjects. While a number of different individually administered IQ tests had previously revealed scores which fell within the normal range, detailed IQ information was not available. All children had been referred by a physician for evaluation in response to evidence of perceptual-motor or educational difficulties, or both.

Testing

Standardized procedures for administering the SCPNT[9] were employed, and 27 children with shorter nystagmus durations ($\bar{X}$ duration = 5.98 sec., S.D. = 3.94) were placed in the Low Nystagmus Group while the remaining 25 children comprised the Comparison Nystagmus Group ($\bar{X}$ duration = 20.76, S.D. = 7.84). The HFD of each child was scored by using the rating scale reported by Ayres and Reid,[11] and it was employed because these researchers found it to be a sensitive measure of the effects of perceptual-motor dysfunction on HFD performance. This scale, which analyzes many of the same characteristics as other rating systems,[e.g., 12] assesses the overall accuracy and detail of human figure drawings and yields a total score that can range from -18 to $+13$. Evaluation of each figure was accomplished independently by two students trained in the scoring system but unfamiliar with the children, their group placement, and the hypothesis. The students compared their evaluations, and where disagreements occurred, they attempted to reach accord through discussion. If they continued to disagree, the first author, also unaware of group placement at the time, made a decision as to which score was correct. The reliability of this procedure was documented (r = .91) by having a third student independently rate the drawings. An analysis of covariance was used to examine drawing scores with age serving as the covariate.

RESULTS

Overall, the two groups did not differ significantly in age [$t(50) = -.58$, $p > .50$] with the Low Nystagmus subjects ($\bar{X} = 90.3$ mo., S.D. = 22.1) slightly younger than the Comparison Nystagmus children ($\bar{X} = 94.0$ mo., S.D. = 23.3). Age, however, was an important determinant of performance [$F(1,49) = 33.02$, $p < .01$], a finding which reflected the improved skill of the older subjects. The analysis of covariance further revealed a significant nystagmus grouping effect [$F(1,49) = 6.40$, $p < .025$] with the drawings of Low children rated lower ($\bar{X} = -4.70$, S.D. = 5.59) than those of the Comparison subjects ($\bar{X} = -0.68$, S.D. = 6.63).

DISCUSSION

In this investigation, children assessed for learning disabilities and perceptual-motor dysfunction were categorized according to the duration of their postrotary nystagmus, and subjects with the shorter durations sketched human figure drawings that were of inferior quality when compared to those drawn by children with relatively longer durations. A possible explanation of these data may be found in the attempt of De-Quiros and Schrager[3] to identify a specific learning disability which they term the "vestibular-oculomotor split." They claim that such a condition can be uncovered through examination of nystagmus and that it can result in "disturbances in ocular fixation and in skilled movements of the eyes." Children with hyporesponsive nystagmus could thus be handicapped in their attempts to integrate ocular movements with hand movements during drawing performance.

Such an explanation is speculative, and additional research into the issue is needed. In particular, future investigations will need to control for the possible confounding effects of factors previously found to be related to HFD skill. For example, IQ scores are positively correlated with figure drawing ability.[13] Therefore, the PRN-HFD association theoretically could have resulted from a sampling error in which children with lower IQ scores were more often placed in the Low Group. In such a situation, the significant grouping effect could have reflected differences in IQ rather than differences in vestibular-proprioceptive functioning. Other variables, including socioeconomic status, have been found to influence HFD performance,[14] and studies controlling these factors will also have to be conducted before definitive conclusions can be reached.

In addition to examining possible confounding variables, subsequent investigations will need to broaden the analysis of vestibular-proprioceptive functioning. Research suggests that abnormally long postrotary nystagmus durations are also indicative of neuropsychological impairment.[2,15] A large group of children with excessively long nystagmus durations was not available for analysis in this project, but the hypothesis that such children would be disadvantaged in their figure drawing ability remains plausible and needs to be tested.

In conclusion, the data presented in this study strengthen the idea that the vestibular characteristics of some learning disabled children are of importance in understanding their difficulties. They also suggest that teachers and other professionals concerned with the educational progress of these students some day may be able to use figure drawings as very gross screening devices for identifying possible specific neuropsychological deficits. As mentioned, however, much more research is needed before this possibility can be realized.

REFERENCES

1. Ayres AJ: *Sensory Integration and Learning Disorders*. Los Angeles, Western Psychological Services, 1972.
2. Ayres AJ: Learning disabilities and the vestibular system. *J Learn Disabil* 11: 30-41, 1978.
3. DeQuiros JB, Schrager O: *Neuropsychological Fundamentals in Learning Disabilities*. San Rafael, CA, Academic Therapy, 1978.
4. Frank J, Levinson H: Dysmetric dyslexia and dyspraxia. *Acad Ther* 11: 133-143, 1975-76.
5. Ottenbacher K: Identifying vestibular processing dysfunction in learning disabled children. *AJOT* 32: 217-221, 1978.
6. Ottenbacher K, Watson PJ, Short MA, Biderman MD: Nystagmus and ocular fixation difficulties in learning disabled children. *AJOT* 33: 717-721, 1978.
7. Ottenbacher K, Short MA, Watson PJ: The use of selected clinical observations to predict postrotary nystagmus change in learning disabled children. *Phys Occup Ther Ped* 1: 31-38, 1980.
8. Swenson CH: Empirical evaluations of human figure drawings: 1957-1966. *Psychol Bull* 70: 20-44, 1968.
9. Ayres AJ: *Southern California Postrotary Nystagmus Test*. Los Angeles, Western Psychological Services, 1972.
10. Culp RE, Packard VN, Humphrey R: Sensorimotor versus cognitive perceptual training effects on the body concept of preschoolers. *AJOT* 34: 259-262, 1980.
11. Ayres AJ, Reid W: The self-drawing as an expression of perceptual motor dysfunction. *Cortex* 2: 254-265, 1966.
12. Harris DB: *Goodenough-Harris Drawing Test Manual*. New York: Harcourt Brace Jovanovich, Inc., 1963.
13. Pikulski JJ: A comparison of figure drawings and WISC IQ's among disabled readers. *J Learn Disabil* 5(3): 41-44, 1972.
14. Scott LH: Measuring intelligence with the Goodenough-Harris Drawing Test. *Psych Bull* 89: 483-505, 1981.
15. Ottenbacher K: Excessive postrotary nystagmus duration in learning-disabled children. *AJOT* 34: 40-44, 1980.

Patterns of Postrotary Nystagmus in Three Learning-Disabled Children

Kenneth Ottenbacher

ABSTRACT. This study explores the effect of a program of sensory integration therapy, with emphasis on vestibular stimulation activities, on the duration of postrotary nystagmus in three learning-disabled children. The single-subject methodology employed allowed a more individualistic and longitudinal investigation of nystagmus patterns in the three subjects. The graphic and statistical analysis of the data revealed that two of the three subjects evidenced significant changes in postrotary nystagmus durations over the 25-week period of the study. Subject 1, with initially low nystagmus durations, displayed an increase in duration, whereas subject 2, with initially normal postrotary nystagmus durations, exhibited a response decline in nystagmus durations. The postrotary nystagmus durations of subject 2 remained relatively stable across both the baseline and intervention periods. The therapeutic implications of the findings are discussed, and areas in need of additional investigation are highlighted.

Recent research has emphasized the importance of testing vestibular and proprioceptive functions when evaluating the neuropsychological attributes of learning-disabled children. Several investigators have demonstrated that significant numbers of children identified as learning disabled or as having minimal brain dysfunction evidence reduced durations of vestibular nystagmus following rotatory stimulation.[1-4] The vestibular ocular reflex being evaluated, postrotary nystagmus (PRN), is a normal physiological response to rotatory vestibular stimulation.[5]

Ayres demonstrated that learning-disabled children with reduced PRN appear to be more responsive to programs of sensory integrative therapy in conjunction with special education than learning-disabled children with normal or hyperresponsive PRN.[1] Ayres developed and standardized a clinical test of PRN that is widely used by therapists to assess the integrity of vestibular ocular reflex function in children.[6] Studies of the Southern California Postrotary Nystagmus Test (SCPNT) have compared the SCPNT with more sophisticated measures of vestibular ocular reflex function and have examined the reliability of the test.[7] These investigations have demonstrated that PRN scores from the SCPNT are correlated with electronystagmographic recording[8] and that PRN durations appear to remain relatively stable. For example, Kimball[9] tested the stability of SCPNT scores over a period of approximately 2 1/2 years and reported a re-test correlation of .80. Recently, Deitz, Siegner, and Crowe[10] found the test/re-test reliability of the SCPNT for 4-year-old children over a 5-week period to be .83.

Ayres[11] originally hypothesized that "the gradual appearance of nystagmus and dizziness from vestibular stimulation is assumed to be an indication that dormant pathways are beginning to be used and may then be available for other sensory integrative processes." (p 119) Ayres and Heskett[12] reported a case study of a young schizophrenic girl receiving sensory integration therapy. The results of the study indicated that therapy had facilitated an increase in PRN duration in the subject. Ottenbacher, Short, and Watson[13] documented changes in PRN for some learning-disabled children receiving sensory integrative therapy. More recently, they[14] reported that, by evaluating specific variables and abilities previously found to be associated with low SCPNT scores, it was possible to predict, to some extent, which learning-disabled children with low PRN durations would respond with PRN increases as the result of therapy and which children would not.

These studies suggested that sensory integrative therapy, employing vestibular stimulation activities, may result in changes in PRN durations; however, the studies to date have not explicated the exact nature of these PRN duration changes. Most of the previous research in this area consisted of comparing treatment and control groups at one or two points in time. In order to investigate the exact nature of PRN duration changes, a more individualistic and longitudinal approach is required.

The purpose of the present study was to examine the effect of a program of sensory integration therapy employing vestibular stimulation activities on the PRN durations of individual learning-disabled children. It was hypothesized that learning-disabled children with low PRN durations (less than -1.0 SD on the SCPNT) would evidence a gradual increase in PRN within the period of the study. It was also hypothesized that learning-disabled children with normal duration PRN would demonstrate a gradual reduction in PRN durations as a result of exposure to repeated vestibular stimulation activities. This hypothesis was based on the large body of literature demonstrating that individuals with normal vestibular ocular reflexes who are repeatedly exposed to vestibular stimulation gradually habituate or adapt to that stimulation through visual fixation and are able to suppress their PRN durations. This normal habituation process has been demonstrated repeatedly in the adult population (i.e., with gymnasts, divers, figure skaters, etc.),[15,16] and has also been reported in learning-disabled children with originally normal duration PRN.[13,14]

SUBJECTS AND METHODS

Three subjects participated in the study. They were Caucasian males enrolled in public school and receiving resource room assistance in at least one academic subject area. The three subjects were identified as learning disabled by school personnel that included a school psychologist and certified learning-disabilities teacher. Each subject was administered a series of evaluative tests. The results of these tests and other relevant descriptive information for each child appear in Table 1.

Postrotary nystagmus durations were recorded twice a week for a period of 25 weeks. The SCPNT was used to obtain the PRN measures and was administered per the standardized instructions. An attempt was made to administer the test at the same time and on the same days each week (Tuesday and Thursday). However, because of illness and school holidays, this was not always possible. The total number of test administrations for each child appears in Table 1.

During the first 5 weeks of the study, the three children did not receive any therapy program. This period served as the baseline. Beginning in the sixth week each child began a program of sensory integrative therapy. Therapy sessions lasted approximately 50 minutes and were conducted three times per week by a therapist experienced in pediatric occupational therapy. The sensory integrative therapy consisted of planned activities designed to enhance the function and integration of the vestibular, proprioceptive, and tactile systems. Treatment was administered to all three subjects during the same period. The emphasis during therapy was on vestibular-proprioceptive activities. These activities stressed passive and active rotatory and linear motion and included rolling games and the use of a sit-and-spin, suspended net hammock, and swings. A variety of scooter board activities were also employed. The children were generally allowed to choose alternately among the activities until all children had participated in all of the activities. The study lasted for a total of 25 weeks—5 weeks of baseline and 20 weeks of intervention.

RESULTS

The weekly average PRN duration for each child was computed and graphed (see Figures 1, 2, and 3). The graphic information clearly demonstrates that changes in PRN durations occurred for two of the three subjects. Subject 1 evidenced an increase in PRN duration during the period of the study. His average baseline PRN duration was 3.5 seconds, whereas his average PRN duration for the last week of the study was 12 seconds. Subject 2 also demonstrated an initially low PRN duration; however, his PRN responses remained relatively stable over the entire

Table 1
Evaluative and Descriptive Information for the Three Subjects

	Subject One	Subject Two	Subject Three
Age (Years)	8.2	7.8	8.6
WISC-R Full Scale IQ	118	92	96
PPVT IQ	110	83	91
SCSIT Scores			
Space Visualization	+0.1	−1.4	−2.4
Figure Ground	+0.9	+0.6	−1.3
Position in Space	−0.7	−1.2	−1.9
Kinesthesia	−1.4	+.02	+0.3
Manual Form Perception	−1.0	−0.1	−2.7
Finger Identification	−1.3	−0.5	−0.6
Graphesthesia	−2.1	−1.7	−1.5
Localization of			
Tactile Stimulation	−0.8	+0.8	−0.4
Double Tactile			
Stimulation	−0.5	−2.1	+0.8
Imitation of Postures	−1.9	−0.9	+0.1
Crossing Midline: Left	−1.6	−2.4	+0.3
Crossing Midline: Right	−1.1	−0.8	+0.1
Bilateral Motor			
Coordination	−1.5	−2.1	−0.1
Right Left Discrimination	−0.9	−2.6	−0.8
Standing Balance: Open	−1.1	−0.7	−0.4
Standing Balance: Closed	−1.9	−0.5	−1.1
Motor Accuracy: Left	−2.4	−2.2	0.0
Motor Accuracy: Right	−2.0	−1.3	+0.6
Design Copy	−1.3	+0.4	−2.1
Clinical Observations*			
Hand Dominance	Right	Right	Right
Eye Dominance	Right	Left	Right
Foot Dominance	Right	Right	Right
Ocular Tracking	Midline Jerk	Midline Jerk	Normal
Muscle Tone	Hypotonic	Normal	Normal
Cocontraction Ability	Fair	Fair	Normal
Flexion Supine Posture	Normal	Normal	Fair
Prone Extension Posture	Poor	Fair	Poor
ATNR Inhibiting Posture	Fair	Poor	Normal
Total SCPNT			
Administrations	44	46	43

*Clinical observations were scored on a 3-point scale with 1 = Poor and 3 = Normal.

baseline and treatment period. His mean PRN duration for the baseline period was 8.6 seconds, whereas his mean PRN duration for the last week of intervention was 10 seconds. Finally, subject 3 evidenced the expected habituation and resultant decline in PRN durations within the 25-week period of the study. Subject 3's mean baseline PRN was 18.8 seconds,

Figure 1

Mean weekly postrotary nystagmus responses for subject one

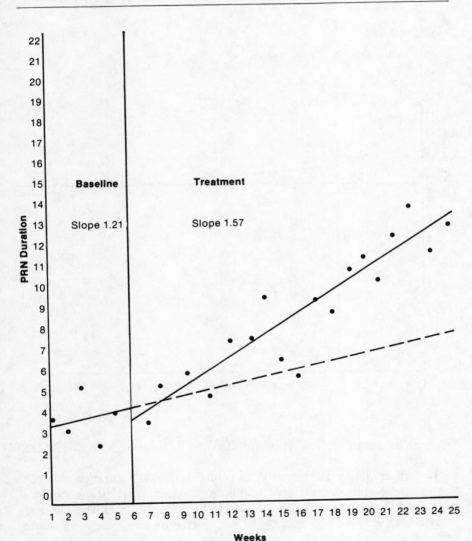

Figure 2
Mean weekly postrotary nystagmus responses for subject two

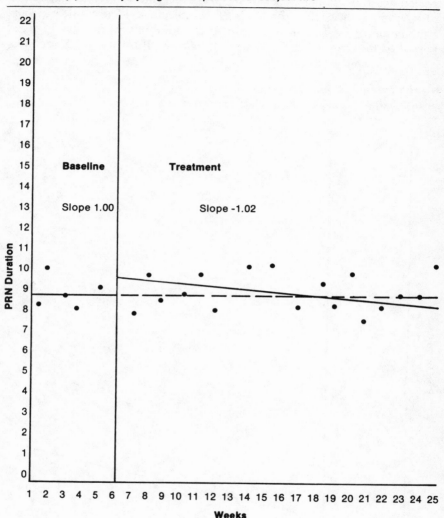

whereas his mean PRN duration for the final week of the study was 11.5 seconds.

To further clarify and quantify the nature of the PRN duration changes for the three subjects, the split middle method of trend estimation was computed for responses from each subject.[17] The split middle technique provides a method of describing the rate of change over time for a single individual. The first step is to plot the data points as shown in the Figures.

Once the data are plotted, the slope or "line of progress" is estimated. The line of progress points in the direction of behavior change and indicates the rate of change. This line is also referred to as the "celeration line," a term derived from the notion of acceleration (if the line of progress is ascending) and deceleration (if the line of progress is descending). Kazdin[17] and White[18] detail the calculation of celeration lines.

Figure 3
Mean weekly postrotary nystagmus responses for subject three

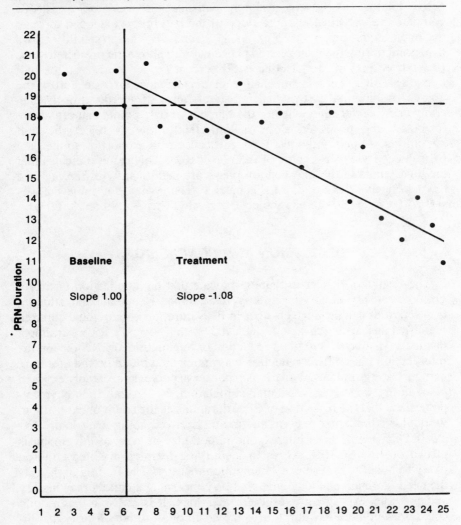

The celeration lines for each phase of the study are included in the figure representing that subject's response pattern. The slope of the individual celeration lines was computed using procedures described by White.[18] The slope merely indicates the rate of change for a particular phase. The change across phases can then be evaluated by comparing the levels and slopes of the celeration lines for the baseline and intervention phases. The slopes for each of the phases for each subject appear in their respective Figures.

To determine whether a statistically significant change in behaviors across phases was present, a simple statistical test was employed.[17] To compute the statistical test, the slope of the baseline is extended through the intervention phase (see Figures 1, 2, and 3). The probability that a data point during the intervention phase will fall above the projected slope (celeration line) of the baseline is 50 percent ($p = .50$), given the null hypothesis that there is no change in performance or rate across the phases. A binomial test or test for significance of a proportion is then computed to determine whether the number of data points that are above or below the projected slope is sufficiently low to reject the null hypothesis. Applying the test for significance of a proportion to the data for subject 1 yields a z value of 2.53 ($p < .02$). This result indicates that the data points in the intervention phase are significantly different from the data during the baseline for subject 1. The z value for subject 2 was -0.24 ($p = .81$), whereas subject 3's z value was -2.99 ($p < .003$).

DISCUSSION AND CONCLUSIONS

The results of this investigation indicate that the application of a program of sensory integration therapy that emphasizes vestibular stimulation activities can produce changes in PRN duration in individual children identified as learning disabled. Subject 3, with "normal" PRN durations, originally displayed a gradual reduction or habituation of PRN during the intervention phase. This reduction was anticipated based on the literature demonstrating similar habituation responses in persons repeatedly exposed to naturally occurring vestibular stimulation.[15, 16] Authorities have hypothesized that the reduction of PRN durations as the result of exposure to vestibular stimulation may be due to an improved ability to visually fixate.[15] This finding is of interest and importance in view of the emphasis placed on low SCPNT scores in identifying learning-disabled children likely to benefit from sensory integration therapy. The finding highlights the need to obtain adequate information concerning a child's play history and previous exposure to vestibular activities. It is possible that a child could present low PRN duration as the result of an activity history that included a good deal of vestibular activity (such as regular play on a sit-and-spin). This child may have developed the ability to visually fixate during rotatory activities and thus exhibit low PRN durations when tested with the SCPNT. A therapist unaware of such a child's previous play history may mistakenly conclude that the low PRN durations are indicative of a vestibular-related dysfunction and not the result of natural PRN habituation from previous exposure to vestibular activities.

The habituation phenomenon may have been partially responsible for the lack of change in subject 2's PRN duration. Subject 2 evidenced low PRN during both the baseline and the intervention periods of the study. The slopes of the celeration lines for subject 2 indicate very little change across phases. Numerous factors have been found to effect PRN duration including degree of mental alertness,[19] visual fixation ability,[20] eye closure,[21] and head position.[22] It is impossible to determine why subject 2 did not respond to intervention with changes in PRN duration; however, it is interesting to note that other measures previously shown to be related to vestibular function[4] were within a normal range for this subject (see Table 1). Ottenbacher, Short, and Watson[14] have shown that, by evaluating these responses associated with vestibular function (i.e., standing balance, pivot prone posture, muscle tone, and cocontraction ability), the ability to "predict" which children with initially low PRN will show increases in PRN duration as a result of therapy is improved. However, it should be noted that Ottenbacher et al. did find some children with normal scores on vestibular-related measures and low PRN durations who did evidence PRN duration increases, and some children with low scores on vestibular-related measures and low initial PRN durations who showed no increase in PRN as the result of therapy.[13, 14]

Subject 1 evidenced the most interesting change in PRN durations during the period of the study. The slopes of the celeration lines for subject 1 indicate a significant increase in PRN duration during the intervention phase. This increase suggests that sensory integration therapy that emphasizes vestibular activities can produce changes in vestibular ocular responses in selected learning-disabled children. The exact mechanism responsible for such change is unclear and is an area in need of further research.

This study provides suggestive support for the theory that the application of controlled sensory stimulation can produce measurable changes in neurovestibular responses; however, the limitations of this investigation should also be considered. The single-subject design employed permits the researcher to study the behavior of individuals over successive observations as opposed to comparing the means of two independent groups of subjects. With such a design it is possible to employ time series measurements or observations and for the subject to serve as his or her own control.[23] The primary disadvantage of single-subject designs is the inability to infer or generalize the results.

Graphic presentation is the traditional analytic tool most frequently used to present the results of single-subject time series designs.[24] Some authorities[25] feel it is not appropriate to employ statistical procedures to applied behavioral or single-subject designs. Elasfoff and Thoresen[26] suggest that visual and statistical analysis should be partners in evaluating the results of single-subject research. That approach was adopted for this investigation.

This study has provided few "conclusions," but has suggested "indications" for future research. The next logical step in this line of investigation would be to explore the relationship between changes in PRN duration and other measures of performance. For example, is an increase in PRN duration associated with improvements in motor function, reflex integration, ocular control, eye-head coordination, and/or improvement in selected academic areas? Also, what are the effects of therapy with children who display response patterns such as those evidenced by subjects 2 and 3? Are subjects with PRN patterns similar to those of subject 2 false positives who will not benefit from therapy? If they are false positives, how can they best be identified so that time, money, and therapeutic efforts are not spent needlessly? Finally, therapists need to develop an awareness or sensitivity to a child's play history so that children with physiologically normal but low PRN are not improperly identified as having a vestibular-related dysfunction on the basis of low PRN durations.

Continued research is needed to delineate the behavioral parameters associated with various PRN response patterns described in this study.

REFERENCES

1. Ayres AJ: Learning disabilities and the vestibular system. *J. Learn Disabil* 11: 30-41, 1978

2. deQuiros JB: Diagnosis of vestibular disorders in the learning disabled. *J. Learn Disabil* 9: 50-58, 1976

3. Steinberg M, Rendle-Short J: Vestibular dysfunction in young children with minor neurological impairment. *Dev Med Child Neurol* 19: 639-651, 1977

4. Ottenbacher K: Identifying vestibular processing dysfunction in learning-disabled children. *Am J Occup Ther* 32: 217-221, 1978

5. Nauton R. (Editor): *The Vestibular System*, New York: Academic Press, 1975

6. Ayres AJ: *Southern California Postrotary Nystagmus Test Manual*, Los Angeles, CA: Western Psychological Corp., 1975

7. Royeen CB: Factors affecting test-retest reliability of the Southern California Postrotary Nystagmus Test. *Am J Occup Ther* 34: 37-39, 1980

8. Keating NR: A comparison of duration of nystagmus as measured by the Southern California Postrotary Nystagmus Test and electronystagmography. *Am J Occup Ther* 33: 92-97, 1972

9. Kimball JG: The Southern California Postrotary Nystagmus Test: Stability over time. In *Integration Topics: Faculty Reviews*, N Tyler, Editor, Los Angeles, CA: CSSID Publication, 1980

10. Deitz JC, Siegner CB, Crowe TK: The Southern California Postrotary Nystagmus Test: Test-retest reliability for preschool children. *Occup Ther J Res* 1: 165-177, 1981

11. Ayres AJ: *Sensory Integration and Learning Disorders*, Los Angeles, CA: Western Psychological Corp., 1972

12. Ayres AJ, Heskett W: Sensory integrative dysfunction in a young schizophrenic girl. *J. Autism Child Schiz* 2: 174-181, 1972

13. Ottenbacher K, Short MA, Watson PJ: Nystagmus duration changes of learning disabled children during sensory integration therapy. *Percept Mot Skill* 48: 1159-1164, 1979

14. Ottenbacher K, Short MA, Watson PJ: The use of selected clinical observations to predict postrotary nystagmus changes in learning disabled children. *Phys Occup Ther Pediatr* 1:31-38, 1980

15. Crampton GH: Habituation of ocular nystagmus of vestibular origin. In *The Oculomotor System*, M. Bender, Editor. New York: Harper & Row, 1964

16. Johnson D, Torok N: Habituation of nystagmus and sensation of motion after rotation. *Acta Otolaryngol* 69: 206-215, 1970

17. Kazdin AE: Statistical analyses for single case experimental designs. In *Single Case Experimental Designs, M. Herson, D. Barlow, Editors*. New York: Pergamon Press, 1976

18. White OR: The split middle a "quickie" method of trend estimation. Experimental Education Unit, Child Development and Mental Retardation Center, University of Washington, 1974

19. Montgomery PC, Capps MJ: Effect of arousal on nystagmus response of normal children. *Phys Occup Ther Pediatr* 1: 17-30, 1980

20. Levy DL, Proctor LR, Holzman PS: Visual interference on vestibular response. *Arch Otolaryngol* 103: 287-291, 1977

21. Tjernstrom O: Nystagmus inhibition as an effect of eye closure. *Acta Otolaryngol* 75: 408-418, 1973

22. Fukuda T: Postural behavior and motion sickness. *Acta Otolaryngol* 81: 237-241, 1976

23. Kratochwill T (Editor): *Single Subject Research: Strategies for Evaluating Change,* New York: Academic Press, 1978

24. Parsonson BS, Baer DM: The analysis and presentation of graphic data. In *Single Subject Research: Strategies for Evaluating Change,* T. Kratochwill, Editor. New York: Acadmic Press, 1978

25. Michael J: Statistical inference for individual organism research: Mixed blessing or curse. *J. Appl Behav Anal* 7: 647-653, 1974

26. Elashoff JD, Thoresen CE: Choosing a statistical method for analysis of an intensive experiment. In *Single Subject Research: Strategies for Evaluating Change,* T. Kratochwill, Editor. New York: Acadmic Press, 1978

Nystagmus Duration Changes of Learning-Disabled Children During Sensory Integrative Therapy

Kenneth Ottenbacher
Margaret A. Short
P. J. Watson

ABSTRACT. Sensory integrative therapy was administered to 43 learning disabled children categorized according to their pretherapeutic duration of postrotary nystagmus. The duration then was recorded after relatively short or long treatments. Children displaying initial subnormal nystagmic functioning responded to therapy with increases in duration while others displayed decreases, and these effects were more apparent after long therapy. These data support the claims that learning disabled children can be meaningfully categorized according to their nystagmic responses and that attention to their interoceptive sensory functioning may be of clinical significance.

A large proportion of learning disabled children evidence vestibular-proprioceptive dysfunction as indicated by poor postural reactions, reduced or abnormal vestibular nystagmic responses, and muscle hypotonicity (Ayres, 1969, 1972; DeQuiros, 1976; Ottenbacher, 1978). Both Ayres (1972) and DeQuiros (1976) have argued that in some learning disabled children these vestibular-proprioceptive deficiencies may contribute to educational difficulties and that attempts at remediation and prevention must address such interoceptive sensory deficits. This study sought to strengthen the empirical foundations for the claim that the duration of postrotary nystagmus of different subgroups of learning disabled children is differentially affected by therapeutic intervention. Of principal interest was the clinical observation of Ayres (1972) that vestibular stimulation gradually produces the nystagmus response in learning disabled children with initially low postrotary nystagmus. Children in this study underwent long-term sensory integrative therapy, a treatment modality that gives patients increased sensory experience in general and increased vestibular-proprioceptive stimulation in particular. An attempt also was made to examine the possibility that the changes in postrotary nystagmus are made more manifest with increasing experience in therapy. This was accomplished by comparing the postrotary nystagmus of children given therapy for a relatively short period of time with the postrotary nystagmus of those who had undergone therapy for a relatively long period.

METHOD

All children attended a children's rehabilitation center to which they had been referred by medical or educational personnel. All had been assessed as learning disabled because their school performances were not commensurate with intellectual potentials. None exhibited overt physical or mental handicaps, and IQs were within normal limits. Ages at the time of initial evaluation ranged from 51 to 125 mo.

Upon referral, each child was administered an extensive evaluation which included the Southern California Postrotary Nystagmus Test, an instrument introduced by Ayres (1975). The standarized procedures were employed by two experienced therapists; and for the present study, the children were divided into three separate groups depending upon their initial response to the nystagmus test. Those children whose duration of postrotary nystagmus was either greater than or less than one standard deviation from the standardized mean on the initial test were placed in the high or the low groups, respectively. Children within one standard deviation above or below the mean were placed in the medium group.

Subjects next were divided into long and short therapy based on criteria of frequency and duration of attendance. The children receiving therapy for at least 6 mo. and attending with a frequency of at least 5 hr. per month for 4 consective mo. were in long therapy. Children not meeting this criterion were said to be in short therapy. So, six groups of subjects were formed, varying both in their initial nystagmic response and in their length of therapeutic experience. Analysis involved examination of initial "pretherapy" nystagmic scores which were taken from the admission score on the nystagmic test and of "posttherapy" nystagmic scores. These latter values represented the average of the last three nystagmic measures acquired for each child in the final stages.

RESULTS

The data are reviewed in Table 1. Pre- and post-therapy durations of nystagmus are relevant to the idea that these subgroups responded differentially during sensory integrative therapy. The children with low initial scores displayed a near doubling of duration of nystagmus after long therapy while subjects with medium and high nystagmus exhibited a decline. An attempt was made to characterize changes in duration over time by computing trend scores. These values were determined by dividing each subject's post-therapeutic duration of nystagmus by the sum of the durations at pre- and post-therapy. Any value over .50 indicated an increase in duration during therapy; and as Table 1 shows, only subjects with initial low nystagmus and who were in therapy for a relatively long interval showed such an effect. These findings are consistent with the contention of Ayres that therapy involving vestibular stimulation can increase postrotary nystagmus in some learning disabled children. Finally, the fact that trend scores for the various groups were farther from .50 after long therapy than after short therapy supports the hypothesis that the effects of therapy increased with time.

Unequal N analyses of variance confirmed the conclusions suggested by the descriptive information. The differential responsiveness of the subgroups to therapy was indicated by a significant effect of nystagmic grouping on the trend scores ($F_{2,37} = 24.81, p < .001$). The significant interaction of nystagmic grouping and length of therapy on the trend scores $F_{2,37} = 5.52, p < .01$) further emphasized the operation of different processes in the nystagmic groups by indicating group-specific changes in duration with the passage of time in therapy. Additional support for this conclusion was obtained with a significant interaction of nystagmus and length of therapy using the duration data ($F_{2,37} = 7.36, p < .01$). Both interactions strengthen the argument that length of time in therapy was important in determining nystagmus duration in the subgroups.

Ethical constraints prevented the withholding of therapy from anyone; therefore, controls for the passage of time could not be utilized. This leaves open the possibility that the alterations in nystagmic duration resulted from maturational processes independent of therapy. At least

TABLE 1

DATA OBTAINED FROM CHILDREN WITH LOW, MEDIUM, OR HIGH NYSTAGMUS
FOLLOWING SHORT OR LONG PERIODS OF THERAPY

		Short Therapy			Long Therapy		
		Low	Medium	High	Low	Medium	High
No. of Children		6	3	3	14	11	6
Age, mo.	M	80.0	75.7	79.0	75.3	73.8	79.8
	σ	24.2	11.7	10.1	13.6	13.1	26.1
Duration of Therapy, mo.	M	4.7	6.0	4.0	9.9	13.3	21.8
	σ	1.8	2.2	0.8	5.8	4.5	5.2
Nystagmus, in sec.							
Pre-therapy	M	5.3	23.0	33.3	5.4	22.5	34.7
	σ	1.7	3.6	1.7	4.2	2.7	5.6
Post-therapy	M	5.4	18.6	21.3	10.2	10.1	8.6
	σ	2.8	10.7	10.8	4.5	5.8	6.3
Trend Score*	M	.48	.41	.37	.71	.29	.18
	σ	.16	.12	.11	.22	.13	.10

*A trend score for each subject was computed by dividing the post-therapy nystagmus duration by the sum of the pre- and post-therapy durations.

three arguments can be made against this alternative explanation. First, there were no significant differences between groups in age, suggesting relatively constant physical maturation across groups. Second, if maturational processes did change duration, then evidence of those processes probably would have been obtained in the pre-therapy duration. In other words, if maturation lengthened duration in subjects with low nystagmus, older children with low nystagmus at the beginning of therapy should have had longer durations than the younger ones. The maturational hypothesis also would have predicted that older children with medium and high nystagmus would have had shorter durations of nystagmus than younger children in these groups. However, no significant correlation was obtained between the age in months and the pre-therapy duration of nystagmus of the children with low nystagmus ($r = .05, p > .10$) or of those with medium and high nystagmus ($r = .26 p > .10$). Finally, Tibbling (1969) reported that pre-rotary durations of nystagmus for normal children from 1 yr. to 15 yr. of age remained fairly stable, suggesting that duration of nystagmus is not sensitive to maturational processes.

However, the length of time in therapy did present one interpretative difficulty because subjects with high nystagmus received significantly longer periods of therapy ($p < .05$, Duncan's range test). It was asked if the observed differences in duration of nystagmus reflected different amounts of time in therapy rather than group-specific responses during the sensory-integrative treatment. A number of points strongly suggest that different processes were in fact operating in the subgroups and that the length of therapy could not be used to explain the pattern of changes in duration. First, groups low and medium in nystagmus did not differ in length of therapy while they displayed opposite changes in duration of nystagmus. Second, examination of what records were available for the subjects with high nystagmus indicated that from the outset their durations declined during therapy. Thus, their "post-therapy" measure was representative of the type of effect observed throughout therapy. Finally, a reduction in the duration of the nystagmic response is typically observed following repeated vestibular stimulation (Crampton, 1964), and the unique aspect of the present data therefore is the increase in duration for the children with low nystagmus. Whether these children given longer therapy continue to display increases, decreases, or level off its presently being examined.

DISCUSSION

These results further strengthen the claims that learning disabled children can be categorized according to characteristics of their post-rotary nystagmus. Children with low nystagmus during sensory integrative therapy exhibited increases in duration while other subjects displayed decreases. In addition, these changes were more apparent following relatively long therapy than relatively short therapy. Correlative evidence suggested that maturational factors were not critical, and length of time in therapy apparently could not be used to explain the observed effects.

In addition, the possibility that the increases in nystagmus represented a regression toward the mean is discounted by two factors. First, research has typically indicated that the normal response to vestibular stimulation is in the direction of decline. Second, it apparently is possible to predict which children with low nystagmus will display an increase in duration during therapy by examining their gross vestibular-proprioceptive functioning.[2] Such a result suggests that increases in duration are not a nonspecific response to therapy nor a statistical artifact.

Although sensory integrative therapy involves a number of components, it may have exerted an influence through increased vestibular-proprioceptive experience. A number of experiments have documented that vestibular-proprioceptive stimulation in infants can enhance motor development (Clark, Kreutzberg, & Chee, 1977), facilitate visual alertness (Gregg, Haffner, & Korner, 1976), and have a soothing effect (Korner & Thoman, 1972). These data may supplement previous demonstrations that vestibular-proprioceptive experience exerts a significant influence on the functioning of physiological and psychological systems.

As mentioned, both DeQuiros and Ayres have argued that treatment of vestibular-proprioceptive dysfunction may be critical in ameliorating the educational difficulties of some learning disabled children. For example, DeQuiros has claimed that children with these deficits must maintain at least some conscious control of vestibular-proprioceptive activities and that this need to attend to interoceptive sensory information interferes with opportunities to accept exteroceptive sensory input. This study has presented suggestive data that sensory integrative therapy may move the functioning characteristics of the vestibular-proprioceptive systems of some learning disabled children toward operational norms.

REFERENCES

Ayres, A. J. Deficits in sensory integration in educationally handicapped children. *Journal of Learning Disabilities,* 1969, 2, 160-168.

Ayres, A. J. *Sensory integration and learning disabilities.* Los Angeles: Western Psychological Services, 1972.

Ayres, A. J. *Southern California postrotary nystagmus test.* Los Angeles: Western Psychological Services, 1975.

Clark, D. L. Kreutzberg, J. R., & Chee, F. K. W. Vestibular stimulation influence on motor development in infants. *Science,* 1977, 196, 1228-1229.

Crampton, G. H. Habituation of ocular nystagmus of vestibular origin. In M. Bender (Ed.), *The oculomotor system.* New York: Harper & Row, 1964. Pp. 332-346.

DeQuiros, J. B. Diagnosis of vestibular disorders in the learning disabled. *Journal of Learning Disabilities,* 1976, 9, 50-58.

Gregg, C. L., Haffner, M. E., & Korner, A. F. The relative efficacy of vestibular-proprioceptive stimulation and the upright position in enhancing visual pursuit in neonates. *Child Development,* 1976, 47, 309-314.

Korner, A. F., & Thoman, E. B. The relative efficacy of contact and vestibular-proprioceptive stimulation in soothing neonates. *Child Development,* 1972, 43, 443-453.

Ottenbacher, K. Identifying vestibular processing dysfunction in learning-disabled children. *American Journal of Occupational Therapy,* 1978, 32, 217-221.

Tibbling, L. The rotary nystagmus response in children. *Acta Oto-Laryngologica,* 1969, 68, 459-467.

Human Figure Drawing Ability and Vestibular Processing Dysfunction in Learning-Disabled Children

Kenneth Ottenbacher
Donna Haley
Carmen Abbott
P. J. Watson

ABSTRACT. Explored the relationship between vestibular function as measured by duration of postrotary nystagmus and human figure drawing ability in 40 children labeled as learning disabled. Regression analysis revealed that the variable of chronological age shared the most variance with human figure drawing scores. Postrotary nystagmus durations also shared a significant amount of variance with human figure drawing scores, while the variables of IQ and sex were nonsignificant. The results provide additional support for the assertion that some learning-disabled children evidence deficits in vestibular processing ability and that these deficits may affect performance on cognitive-perceptual tasks.

Recently, Levinson (1980) postulated that some learning-disabled children evidence signs of a cerebellar-vestibular dysfunction that may interfere with the coordination of eye-head movement and ocular tracking and thus produce specific reading disorders. The assertion that a subgroup in the learning-disabled population is affected by some type of vestibular processing disorder is not new. Ayres (1972) identified a group of learning disabled children characterized by low muscle tone, poor postural adjustment reactions, deficits in ocular tracking, and reduced postrotatory nystagmus after vestibular stimulation. All of these characteristics are suggestive of vestibular-related dysfunction (Ayres, 1978).

deQuiros and Schrager (1978) also have identified vestibular dysfunction in some learning-disabled children. deQuiros (1976) originally referred to a syndrome labeled vestibular-proprioceptive disintegration characterized by muscle hypotonia, poorly integrated postural mechanisms, delays in motor and language development, and reduced or abnormal reactions to neurovestibular testing. deQuiros and Schrager (1978) identified another related syndrome termed vestibular-oculomotor split, which results in impaired ocular fixation and scanning ability and poor eye-head coordination.

111

Both Ayres (1972, 1978) and deQuiros and associates (1976, 1978) repeatedly have found significant numbers of children identified as learning disabled who display depressed or abnormal vestibular-ocular reflexes, referred to as nystagmus, after rotatory or caloric stimulation of the vestibular apparatus. Independent researchers have reported studies that tend to confirm the existence of vestibular related dysfunction in some members of the learning-disabled population. These investigations have shown that some children with learning disabilities display characteristic soft or non-focal neurologic signs (Ottenbacher, 1978; Ottenbacher, Short, & Watson, 1980; Steinberg & Rendle-Short, 1977), and low scores on tests of visual-motor integration, reading achievement, and ocular scanning (Cheek, 1970; Levinson, 1980; Ottenbacher, Watson, Short, & Biderman, 1979).

Recently Watson, Ottenbacher, Short, Kittrell, and Workman (1981) reported that the human figure drawings of children with reduced postrotary nystagmus (PRN) were judged to be significantly less well developed than the human figure drawings produced by learning-disabled children with normal postrotary nystagmus durations. Levinson (1980) has provided examples of learning-disabled children's figure drawings that reflect deficits in cerebellar-vestibular function. Levinson (1980) hypothesized that impaired ocular scanning ability and spatial relation skills related to cerebellar-vestibular dysfunction are partially responsible for the poor figure drawing performance of some learning disabled children with reading disorders. Levinson (1980) states that, "As a result of the insights derived from the c-v [cerebellar-vestibular] mechanisms correlated to normal and dyslexic functioning, it appeared reasonable to view the Goodenough figure performance in terms of neurodynamic projections of the c-v [cerebellar-vestibular] modulated sensory-motor body scheme. Goodenough errors exceeding developmental norms may hereafter be viewed as reflecting the body image distortions resulting from specific patterns of c-v [cerebellar-vestibular] and related CNS and psychogenic dysfunctioning" (p. 58). Culp, Packard, and Humphrey (1980) reported that the human figure drawing performance of preschool children was improved by a sensorimotor program that included attention to vestibular input. Their findings further suggest a linkage between vestibular system functioning and ability to draw human figures.

The general purpose of this investigation was to explore further the relationship of human figure drawing ability and vestibular processing function as measured by postrotary nystagmus. A continued analysis of this issue is necessitated by the fact that numerous extraneous variables correlate with figure drawing performance (Scott, 1981; Swenson, 1968), and the possibility therefore exists that the postrotatory nystagmus—figure drawing relationship is mediated by one or more of these variables. For example, Watson and associates (1981) demonstrated a correlation without access to IQ data, which are associated with drawing skill, and this study specifically sought to determine whether the relationship operates independently of IQ.

METHOD

Subjects

*S*s were 40 children (28 male and 12 female), who ranged in age from 59 to 146 months. A multidisciplinary team identified all *S*s as learning disabled based on the results of several individually administered tests and consultation with teachers and parents. All children were receiving specialized remedial instruction and evidenced IQ scores within the normal range (IQ > 80).

Testing

All *S*s were administered a standardized individual intelligence test by a state licensed examiner. In addition, all *S*s received an exam by a physician and an evaluation of motor and postural function by a physical therapist. Specific children received additional testing related to their individual area of academic, language/learning or perceptual dysfunction. These additional tests were administered by a learning disabilities specialist, a speech/language pathologist, and a physical therapist at a university medical center in a midwestern city.

Measures of postrotary nystagmus (PRN) duration were obtained for each child from the Southern California Postrotary Nystagmus Test (Ayres, 1975). This instrument provides a direct measure of vestibular-ocular reflexes (PRN) in children 5 to 10 years of age. The test is modeled after the Barany procedure, and results of the test have been found to compare favorably with ENG evaluations (Keating, 1979). Detailed validity and reliability information have been reported elsewhere (Ayres, 1975; Deitz, Siegner, & Crowe, 1981; Punwar, 1982; Royeen, 1980). Each child also was requested to draw a picture of him/herself as a part of the evaluation. The human figure drawings for each child were scored blindly using a rating scale reported by Ayres and Reid (1966). The scale was also used by Watson et al. (1981) in their investigation of postrotary nystagmus duration and human figure drawings in learning-disabled children. These investigators found the rating system to be a sensitive measure of the relationship between sensorimotor dysfunction and human drawing performance in learning-disabled children. The rating system assesses the overall accuracy and detail of human figure drawings and yields a total score that ranges from −18 to +13. Evaluation of each child's drawing was accomplished by two raters trained in the scoring system, but unfamiliar with the nature of the study or the hypotheses under investigation. The raters compared their evaluations and attempted to reach accord through discussion. If they continued to disagree, one of the authors (PJW), who was unaware of *S*'s test performance, made a decision as to which score was correct. An interrater reliability of .94 was found for the rating system.

RESULTS

Descriptive information for the sample appears in Table 1.

A regression analysis was performed to investigate the relationship of human figure drawing performance to other variables of interest. In the regression analysis, the human figure drawing score served as the dependent or criterion variable, and the variables of age, IQ, postrotary nystagmus duration, and sex functioned as independent or predictor variables. Sex was coded as a dummy variable. Dummy variable coding was used to render the information regarding membership in one group (male vs. female) by a series of g-1 dichotomies. Variable coding was performed according to Cohen and Cohen (1975). The MaxR squared regression program from the Statistical Analysis System package (SAS Institute, 1979) was employed to generate the regression equations. This procedure selects the best one variable regression model that produces the largest R^3, then the best two, three, and four variable models, respectively. The MaxR squared procedure generally is accepted as superior to more widely used simple stepwise procedures (SAS, 1979). Table 2 includes the correlation matrix for the variables under investigation, while Table 3 presents the four models, the variables included in each step, the R^2 and the corresponding F value. Table 3 indicates that the combination of all four predictor variables (age, PRN, IQ, and sex) produced an R^2 of .384, which indicates that approximately 38.4% of the variance in human figure drawing performance could be accounted for by the four independent variables. Age was the first variable added in the model, postrotary nystagmus duration was second, IQ was third, and sex was added last. The R^2 values indicate that age and postrotary nystagmus duration shared the most variance with human figure drawing scores, while IQ and sex contributed little to the shared variance. (See Tables 2 and 3.)

Further analysis revealed that those *S*s with low postrotary nystagmus durations (less than -1.0 *SD* on the Southern California Postrotary Nystagmus Test) were significantly younger than those *S*s with normal postrotary nystagmus duration ($t(38) = 2.61, p < .05$). There were no significant difference in IQ scores in terms of postrotary nystagmus durations ($t(38) = .73, p < .10$).

TABLE 1

Descriptive Information for the Sample

Male	N	28
Female	N	12
Age	M	87.95
	SD	22.91
IQ	M	93.13
	SD	12.40

TABLE 2

*Correlation Coefficients for Variables
Included in Regression Model*[a]

Variables	PRN	Age	IQ	HFD
PRN	1.0	.42	.11	.49
Age	—	1.0	.27	.52
IQ	—	—	1.0	.26
HFD	—	—	—	1.0

[a]Product-moment correlations were not computed for the categorical variable of sex.

PRN = Postrotary Nystagmus.

HFD = Human Figure Drawing.

TABLE 3

Results of Regression Procedure

Step	Model	R^2	F
1	Human Figure Drawing = Age	.27	14.30*
2	Human Figure Drawing = Age PRN	.37	10.74*
3	Human Figure Drawing = Age PRN IQ	.38	7.49*
4	Human Figure Drawing = Age PRN IQ Sex	.38	5.46*

*$p < .01$.

To investigate the effects of age and postrotary nystagmus duration on human figure drawing, an analysis of covariance was performed. Depressed ($-1,0$ SD) vs. normal postrotary nystagmus durations served as the independent variable, human figure drawing scores served as the dependent measure, and age as the covariate. The analysis revealed an $F(1,37)$ of 5.49 ($p < .025$), which indicates a significant difference in human figure drawing scores based on postrotary nystagmus durations when the variable of age was controlled statistically.

DISCUSSION AND CONCLUSIONS

The results of this study support the contention of previous investigators that some learning-disabled children can be differentiated based on their performance on measures of vestibular-ocular function. This study also suggests that human figure drawing may be used as one indicator of vestibular related dysfunction in some learning-disabled children and that the postrotary nystagmus—figure drawing relationship operates independently of IQ.

The ability to complete human figure drawings depends on the child's age, as was demonstrated by the strong correlation of this variable with figure drawing scores and the importance of the age variable in the regression model. However, age-appropriate human figure drawings also depend upon adequate motor control, eye-hand coordination, and the ability to relate one's body to external space. All of these functions are influenced or moderated in part by the vestibular apparatus (Parker, 1980). The fact that deficits in the processing of vestibular related information may contribute to poor human figure drawing was evidenced by the large variance postrotary nystagmus durations shared with human figure drawing scores. In contrast, IQ, which often is associated with human figure drawing performance, correlated minimally with figure drawing ability.

Schilder (1933) was one of the first investigators to hypothesize the importance of the vestibular system in overall human development. He argued that the vestibular system served an integrating and coordinating function in the central nervous system and played an important role in the development of body image and other related neuropsychological functions. To the extent that human figure drawings are indicators of a learning-disabled child's body image, the results of this investigation offer suggestive support for Schidler's assertion.

In conclusion, the data presented in this study support the hypothesis that vestibular related dysfunction, present in some learning-disabled children, is important in understanding their perceptual and neuropsychological deficits. The results also indicate that human figure drawings in learning-disabled children may reflect possible specific dysfunction related, in part, to the inability to process adequately vestibular related information. Additional research obviously is needed to substantiate such a relationship.

REFERENCES

Ayres, A.J. (1972). *Sensory integration and learning disorders.* Los Angeles: Western Psychological Services.

Ayres, A.J. (1975). *Southern California Postrotary Nystagmus Test.* Los Angeles: Western Psychological Services.

Ayres, A.J. (1978). Learning disabilities and the vestibular system. *Journal of Learning Disabilities*, 12, 18-29.

Ayres, A.J., & Reid, W. (1966). The self-drawing as an expression of perceptual motor dysfunction. *Cortex*, 2, 254-265.

Cheek, C. W. (1970). Electronystagmography in children with specific learning disability. *Dissertation International*, 30, 2171A.

Cohen, J., & Cohen, P. (1975). *Applied multiple regression/correlation analysis for the behavioral sciences*. New York: John Wiley.

Culp, R. E., Packard, V., & Humphrey, R. (1980). Sensorimotor versus cognitive perceptual training effects on the body concept of preschoolers. *American Journal of Occupational Therapy*, 34, 259-262.

Dietz, J. C., Siegner, C. B., & Crowe, T. K. (1981). The Southern California Postrotary Nystagmus Test: Test-retest reliability for school children. *Occupational Therapy Journal of Research*, 2, 165-178.

deQuiros, J. B. (1976). Diagnosis of vestibular disorders in the learning disabled. *Journal of Learning Disabilities*, 9, 50-58.

deQuiros, J. B., & Schrager, O. L. (1978). *Neuropsychological fundamentals in learning disabilities*. San Rafael, CA: Academic Therapy Press.

Keating, N. R. (1979). A comparison of nystagmus duration by the Southern California Postrotary Nystagmus Test and electronystagmography. *American Journal of Occupational Therapy*, 33, 92-97.

Levinson, H. N. (1980). *A solution to the riddle—dyslexia*. New York: Springer-Verlag.

Ottenbacher, K. (1978). Identifying vestibular processing dysfunction in learning disabled children. *American Journal of Occupational Therapy*, 32, 217-221.

Ottenbacher, K., Short, M. A., & Watson, P. J. (1980). The use of selected clinical observations to predict postrotary nystagmus change in learning disabled children. *Physical & Occupational Therapy in Pediatrics*, 1, 31-38.

Ottenbacher, K., Watson, P. J., Short, M. A., & Biderman, M. (1979). Nystagmus and ocular fixation difficulties in learning disabled children. *American Journal of Occupational Therapy*, 33, 717-721.

Parker, D. E. (1980). The vestibular apparatus. *Scientific American*, 243, 118-135.

Punwar, A. (1982). Expanded normative data: Southern California Postrotary Nystagmus Test. *American Journal of Occupational Therapy*. 36, 183-187.

Royeen, C. B. (1980). Factors affecting test-retest reliability of the Southern California Postrotary Nystagmus Test. *American Journal of Occupational Therapy*, 34, 664-670.

SAS Institute (1979). *SAS user's guide*. Cary, NC: SAS Institute.

Schilder, P. (1933). The vestibular apparatus in neurosis and psychosis. *Journal of Nervous and Mental Disease*, 78, 1-23.

Scott, L. H. (1981). Measuring intelligence with the Goodenough-Harris Drawing Test. *Psychological Bulletin*. 89, 483-505.

Steinberg, M., & Rendle-Short, J. (1977). Vestibular dysfunction in young children with minor neurological impairment. *Developmental Medicine and Child Neurology*, 19, 639-651.

Swenson, C. H. (1968). Empirical evaluations of human figure drawings: 1957-1966. *Psychological Bulletin*, 70, 20-44.

Watson, P. J., Ottenbacher, K., Short, M. A., Kittrell, J., & Workman, E. (1981). Human figure drawings of learning disabled children with hyporesponsive postrotary nystagmus. *Physical & Occupational Therapy in Pediatrics*, 1, 21-26.

The Use of Selected
Clinical Observations to Predict
Postrotary Nystagmus Change
in Learning Disabled Children

Kenneth Ottenbacher
Margaret A. Short
P. J. Watson

ABSTRACT. Twenty-six children diagnosed as learning disabled and displaying hyporesponsive postrotary nystagmus were divided on the basis of four measures of vestibular-proprioceptive function commonly employed by therapists to evaluate reflex integration and postural mechanisms. Data analysis revealed that learning disabled children with combined hyporesponsive postrotary nystagmus and associated vestibular-proprioceptive deficits were more likely to evidence increases in postrotary nystagmus durations following sensory integrative therapy. Results are discussed in terms of the relationship between hyporesponsive postrotary nystagmus and clinical measures of vestibular-proprioceptive functions. The possible existence of separate identifiable syndromes of vestibular processing dysfunction and their respective responsiveness to sensory integrative therapy are examined.

A large proportion of learning disabled (LD) children reportedly exhibit vestibular-proprioceptive (V-P) deficiencies characterized by abnormal nystagmus, muscle hypotonicity, and atypical postural responses.[1,3] It recently was suggested that in order to more accurately identify vestibular processing dysfunction, clinical assessments should include evaluation of a constellation of variables.[4] Supporting this argument was the observation that reduced nystagmus in LD children was related to muscle hypotonicity and to an inability to maintain or assume a prone extension posture or standing balance with the eyes open or closed. In addition, LD children with normal or high postrotary nystagmus durations generally demonstrated reductions in this measure during a program of sensory integrative therapy while LD children with suppressed postrotary nystagmus exhibited increases.[5] Such data present further evidence that LD children can be differentiated according to the operating characteristics of their V-P systems.

A close examination of the effects of sensory integrative therapy on nystagmus duration revealed that not all children with initial hyporesponsive nystagmus exhibited subsequent increases in nystagmus duration.[5] Since suppressed nystagmus may result not only from vestibular-proprioceptive processing deficits, but also from a number of other variables such as the presence of light in the visual field,[6] reductions in arousal, or visual fixation,[7] it was decided to further examine the characteristics of these LD-low nystagmus duration children. Specifically, the purpose of the present study was to determine if V-P variables could be used to predict the LD children most likely to respond to therapy with nystagmus duration increases. Based on the suggestion that attention to global V-P functioning is important in accurately assessing interoceptive sensory deficits,[4] it was hypothesized that LD children with low duration nystagmus and with greater V-P deficiency would respond to therapy with greater increases in postrotary nystagmus duration than would other low nystagmus children without such strong evidence of V-P dysfunction. It was hoped that this information would aid the clinician in identifying the low duration nystagmus LD children with vestibular-proprioceptive systems most receptive to sensory integrative therapy.

CHILDREN AND METHOD

The 26 children in this study attended a children's rehabilitation center to which they had been medically referred with a diagnosis of learning disability or perceptual-motor dysfunction. Prior to admission to the rehabilitation center, each child was evaluated with the Southern California Sensory Integration Test (SCSIT), the Southern California Postrotary Nystagmus Test (SCPNT), and an assessment of muscle tone, reflex integration, and postural mechanisms. All evaluations were individually administered by one of two occupational therapists, one of whom was certified in the administration and interpretation of the SCSIT. Following evaluation, each child was placed into a program of sensory integrative therapy.

For inclusion in this study, all children displayed low duration nystagmus by scoring more than one standard deviation below the mean of the initial SCPNT. Data from most of these children (71% of the Low V-P group and 75% of the High V-P group) were taken from the low duration nystagmus group from a previous study exploring a different issue.[5] The additional children had been subsequently referred to the rehabilitation center. To meet criteria for the study, all children additionally were required to attend therapy for at least four months with a minimum of five hourly sessions per month. The nature of this therapy has been previously described in detail.[8]

During the course of therapy, the SCPNT was administered bimonthly to all children. The purpose of continued measurement was to track possible changes in the duration of nystagmus during exposure to sensory integrative therapy. At the time the study was completed, a terminal nystagmus score was computed by averaging the last two scores on the SCPNT. The duration of therapy for all children ranged from five to 24 months. A V-P score was obtained for all children by totaling scores on four measures which were previously demonstrated to be related with low SCPNT scores. These measures were assessed as part of the intake evaluation and before therapy was initiated. The measures and their scoring method are reported in Table 1.

The V-P scores for all children were ranked, and a median score was obtained. All children with scores less than the median of 9 were placed in a Low-V-P group, and all children with a score of 9 or more were placed in a High V-P group. To determine if these two groups differed on the basis of their initial or terminal nystagmus responses, the data were analyzed using a 2×2 (one between-one within) Least Squares Analysis of Variance (ANOVA) for unequal N with the V-P (Low versus High) and test (initial versus terminal) values serving as independent variables and postrotary nystagmus duration as the dependent variable. In addition, the groups were examined for differences in age and duration of therapy.

Table 1

Clinical Measures of Vestibular-Proprioceptive Function

Muscle Tone*	Score
Definitely hypotonic	1
Moderately hypotonic	2
Normal	3
Prone Extension Posture*	
Unable to assume and hold	1
Assume and hold for 0-19 seconds	2
Assume and hold for 20 seconds or more	3
Standing Balance Eyes Closed	
Standard score of -2.0 or less	1
Standard score of -1.0 to -1.9	2
Standard score greater than -1.0	3
Standing Balance Eyes Open	
Standard score of -2.0 or less	1
Standard score of -1.0 to -1.9	2
Standard score greater than -1.0	3

*Methods of measuring these variables have been reported[4]

RESULTS

As Table 2 indicates, 12 children fell in the Low V-P group with 14 in the High V-P group. Of the Low V-P children, all but one exhibited terminal nystagmus scores that were higher than their initial nystagmus duration. On the other hand, of the 14 children in the High V-P group, only one-half had higher terminal nystagmus durations. Further, the Low V-P group exhibited a lower mean initial nystagmus but a higher mean terminal nystagmus duration when compared with the mean initial and terminal nystagmus measures of the High V-P group.

The results of the ANOVA (Table 3) comparing these two groups indicated that there was no significant V-P main effect [$F(1,24) = 1.01$, $p < .20$]; however, a significant Test effect [$F(1,24) = 12.80, p < .005$] and a significant V-P-by-Test interaction [$F(1,24) = 5.37, p < .05$] were obtained. These data indicate that in terms of the overall duration of nystagmus, the groups did not differ; nevertheless, the two groups demonstrated a significant differential nystagmus response to the effects of time in therapy.

In order to clarify the nature of this differential responsiveness, planned comparisons were conducted. The results of these t-tests revealed that in the High V-P group, the initial and terminal nystagmus durations were not significantly different ($t = 1.06$, df = 13, $p > .10$, two tailed), but that in the Low V-P group, the terminal nystagmus duration was sig-

Table 2

Characteristics of the Low and High

Vestibular-Proprioceptive Groups of

LD Children With Depressed PRN

	Low V-P	High V-P
No. of Children	12	14
X̄ Age in mos.	75.4	78.6
(Standard Deviation)	(15.2)	(10.8)
X̄ Duration of Therapy in mos.	9.5	9.1
(Standard Deviation)	(4.8)	(4.9)
X̄ Initial Nystagmus Duration in secs.	5.2	6.6
(Standard Deviation)	(3.7)	(4.0)
X̄ Terminal Nystagmus Duration in secs.	11.8	8.2
(Standard Deviation)	(3.8)	(4.1)

Table 3

Source Table from ANOVA Comparing Nystagmus Duration

of Low and High V-P Subjects (Between Factor)

on Initial and Terminal (Within Factor) Tests

Source	Sum of Squares	Degress of Freedom	Mean Squares	F
Between Subjects	366.70	25		
Between Factor	14.84	1	14.84	1.01
Error Between	351.86	24	14.67	
Within Subjects	659.01	26		
Within Factor	200.08	1	200.08	12.80**
Between x Within Interaction	83.88	1	83.88	5.37*
Error Within	375.05	24	15.63	

* p <.05
** p <.005

nificantly higher than the initial nystagmus measure (t - 4.09, df = 11, p < .01, two tailed). This contrasting responsiveness of the Low and High V-P groups cannot be explained by differences in age or in duration of therapy, since t-tests for unrelated means indicated that there were no significant differences in age (t = .61, df = 24, p > .50, two tailed) nor in duration of therapy (t = .18, df = 24, p > .50, two tailed).

DISCUSSION

The recent research of Ayres has emphasized the importance of differential identification of LD children based on vestibular function as measured by postrotary nystagmus durations.[9] She found that LD children receiving sensory integrative therapy and exhibiting depressed SCPNT scores (< 1lSD) showed significantly greater improvement on academic measures than did LD children with normal or hyperresponsive nystagmus. In addition, other researchers have reported that LD children with depressed nystagmus also may exhibit reduced ocular scanning abilities when compared to LD children with normal nystagmus, and suggestive evidence has been presented indicating that their ocular fixation ability may improve along with increases in nystagmus duration during sensory integrative therapy.[8] Finally, recent analysis has revealed a tentative association between depressed postrotary nystagmus in LD children and the presence of socially inappropriate behaviors, particularly in boys,[10] a finding which further suggests that LD children can be meaningfully categorized according to their nystagmus characteristics.

The data from the present study indicate that different processes may be responsible for the initial reduced nystagmus measures in some LD children. As mentioned, depressed nystagmus may be due not only to dysfunction in vestibular processing ability, but also due to environmental lighting, visual fixation, and reductions in arousal level. It is possible, then, that some LD children exhibit reduced nystagmus, not because of vestibular dysfunction, but due to the effects of such extraneous variables; consequently, these children maintain stable low nystagmus durations despite long-term therapy. Autistic children apparently demonstrate reduced nystagmus duration when tested in a lighted room and normal nystagmus duration when blindfolded.[11] Ritvo and co-workers suggest that these inconsistent measurements reflect disturbances in the regulation of sensory input in emotionally disturbed children. That learning disabled children displaying reduced nystagmus durations may also evidence manifestations of behavioral disorders has been previously suggested.[10]

It should be pointed out that in the group that demonstrated higher scores in vestibular-proprioceptive function as measured by selected clinical observations, one-half of the children who originally displayed hyporesponsive nystagmus durations did show increases in nystagmus duration during therapy. Since these children did not display associated vestibular-proprioceptive deficiencies, it is not clear why they responded with increased durations. One possible explanation is that these children may still possess vestibular deficits which respond to sensory integrative therapy but which are not made manifest through muscle hypotonia, inadequate reflex integration, or abnormal postural responses. The possibility that separate vestibular syndromes produce learning disabilities has been proposed by DeQuiros and Schrager.[12] They have stated that primary learning disabilities are due to a number of clinical abnormalities. One syndrome, termed vestibular-proprioceptive dissociation, is global in nature and is characterized by disturbances in posture, equilibrium, and body movements. The second syndrome, termed vestibular-oculomotor split, is characterized by disturbances of skilled movements of the eyes and produces subsequent reading disabilities.[12(pp107-112)] A similar hypothesis has been proposed by Frank and Levinson,[13] who link dysfunction of the vestibular system, the cerebellum, and the oculomotor system with dyslexia. Thus, the possibility exists that children with apparently normal postural mechanisms and reflex integration but who have initial depressed nystagmus durations that increase during therapy are representative of this latter, vestibular-oculomotor syndrome.

The results of the present study indicate that the therapist may be able to refine and enhance diagnostic and therapeutic procedures by combining global measures of vestibular-proprioceptive and postural responding with the SCPNT. This procedure may facilitate a determination of LD children most likely to demonstrate a normalization of nystagmus responses following exposure to sensory integrative therapy. That therapists should concern themselves with this information assumes that a return of the vestibular ocular reflex system to normal operative parameters is an important therapeutic goal, and Ayres[1,9] has argued cogently that this should be an objective of therapy. However, the behavioral and educational significance of nystagmus duration changes in LD children remains to be fully explicated; further research is obviously needed.

REFERENCES

1. Ayres AJ: *Sensory Integration and Learning Disorders.* Los Angeles, Western Psychological Services, 1972.
2. DeQuiros JB: Diagnosis of vestibular disorders in the learning disabled. *J Learn Disabil* 9:50-58, 1976.
3. Steinberg M, Rendle-Short J: Vestibular dysfunction in young children with minor neurological impairment. *Dev Med Child Neurol* 19:639-651, 1977.
4. Ottenbacher K: Identifying vestibular processing dysfunction in learning disabled children. *AJOT* 32:217-221, 1978.
5. Ottenbacher K, Short MA, Watson PJ: Nystagmus duration changes of learning disabled children during sensory integrative therapy. *Percep Mot Skills* 48:1159-1164, 1979.
6. Levy D, Proctor L, Holzman P: Visual interference on vestibular response. *Arch Otolaryngol* 103:287-291, 1977.
7. Cogan D: *Neurology of the Ocular Muscles*, ed 2. Springfield, IL, Charles C Thomas, 1956.
8. Ottenbacher K, Watson P, Short MA, Biderman MD: Nystagmus and ocular fixation difficulties in learning disabled children. *AJOT* 33:717-721, 1979.
9. Ayres AJ: Learning disabilities and the vestibular system. *J Learn Disabil* 11:30-41, 1978.
10. Ottenbacher K, Watson P, Short MA: Association between nystagmus hyporesponsivity and behavioral problems in learning disabled children. *AJOT* 33:317-322, 1979.
11. Ritvo E, Ornitz E, Eviatar A, et al: Decreased postratary nystagmus in early infantile autism. *Neurol* 19:653-658, 1969.
12. DeQuiros JB, Schrager O: *Neuropsychological Fundamentals in Learning Disabilities.* San Rafael, CA, Academic Therapy, 1978.
13. Frank J, Levinson H: Dysmetric dyslexia and dyspraxia. *Acad Ther* 11:133-143, 1975-76.

PART 5:
EXPERIMENTAL DESIGN
FOR CLINICAL INVESTIGATION

In the studies discussed in the preceding sections of this anthology, a variety of research designs was used. Some designs were used because of the nature of previously collected data, while other designs were used because of the restrictions imposed by time, therapy, or restraints regarding the development of a control group. The final study included in this anthology is an example of a well-developed experimental design used in a clinical setting. As was pointed out in the Introduction to this collection, true experimental and quasi-experimental studies differ primarily in amount of control they are able to exert over variables. Both types of designs specify independent and dependent variables, and both use experimental and control groups. But the quasi-experimental design often does not include the random assignment of subjects. This is the kind of design that is often necessary to use in the clinic.

Experimental designs are used to study cause and effect relationships and are particularly suitable for assessing the effects of particular therapeutic interventions. In true experimental designs subjects are selected randomly, meaning that every single subject with the necessary characteristics to participate in the study, has an equal chance of being selected. Similarly, subjects are randomly assigned to either a treatment or control group; this can be done by picking numbers out of a hat, giving each subject an equal chance of belonging to the treatment or control condition. The true experimental design is difficult to apply in clinical situations. Subjects do not come to the clinic at random—they are referred for specific reasons. Clinical subjects may belong to a particular region of a city or to a particular socioeconomic group, and they may not be at all representative of the population at large. Additionally, a therapist may be restricted by the extent to which a subject can be assigned to a control population (see Ethics, Part 3). Thus, clinical therapists adopt quasi-experimental methodologies, and attempt as much as possible to adhere to rules regarding control or randomization.

One characteristic of a study which demonstrates the effectiveness of a therapeutic intervention is that it follows, as much as possible, the rules for experimental design. It thereby reduces possible confounds by random assignment of subjects, by blind assessment of subjects, and by clearcut design and definition of variables to enable the ease of data analysis and interpretation. Most of these characteristics are exemplified in the study reported in this section. Unfortunately, this study did not include a blind assessor, someone who is unaware of the group assignments of the children. Thus some bias could have been added by unintended cues or interpretations of the examiner. Otherwise, the study is a sound example of clinical experimental research, and it illustrates how more straightforward conclusions can be drawn with this kind of design than with correlational studies (see Part 2).

As we mentioned previously, the results of one study can only be considered tentative. Too many extraneous variables can affect the results of a study, and research is conclusive only when it is considered within a context of an entire body of similar research. This particular study, "The Effects of a Clinically Applied Program of Vestibular Stimulation on the Neuromotor Performance of Children with Severe Developmental Disability" (Reprint 12), is an excellent illustration of this point. This study illustrates that controlled vestibular stimulation, using a regime similar in intensity and duration to one used by other researchers,[1,2] resulted in enhanced motor abilities in developmentally delayed children. These findings are similar to those of Clark and colleagues, but they still are not conclusive. The studies conducted by Clark and his colleagues have been criticized because of the small numbers of subjects and because the procedures were conducted under very controlled experimental conditions that may not be applicable to the clinic. While our study lends support to the conclusions made by Clark and his colleagues, additional research is equivocal. For example, the results of Sellick and Over's[3] investigation of the effects of vestibular stimulation with cerebral palsied children conflict with those of Clark and colleagues and with our findings.

This type of conflict in the literature should not be discouraging to the clinician. First, studies should be regarded in a context; thus, one study is not conclusive. Second, differing results illuminate conditions where intervention may, or may not, be effective. The types of subjects examined by Clark and colleagues, Sellick and Over, and by us are all different—they differed in age, as well as type and severity of disability. Additionally, the test instruments (assessment tools) differed, changing the dependent variables from study to study. Such differences in apparently similar studies point out the need for future studies which will narrow down the variables and may contribute to a body of literature which will eventually determine the specific effects or the scope of certain kinds of vestibular stimulation. This focus on specific target variables is the raison d'être of research, and much of this focus could not occur without multiple studies (which may yield conflicting findings). Readers are strongly encouraged to examine the references that are cited in this section, as well as subsequent examinations of the effects of vestibular stimulation,[4-7] in order to compare and to contrast the different samples, procedures, data analyses and their effects. The introduction to the study by Sellick and Over,[3] in particular, gives an excellent description of the characteristics of rigorous experimental design.

REFERENCES

1. Chee FKW, Kreutzberg JR, Clark DL: Semicircular canal stimulation in cerebral palsied children. *Phys Ther* 58:1071-1075, 1978.

2. Clark DL, Kreutzberg JR, Chee FKW: Vestibular stimulation influence on motor development in infants. *Science* 196:1228-1229, 1977.

3. Sellick KJ, Over R: Effects of vestibular stimulation on motor development of cerebral palsied children. *Dev Med Child Neurol* 11:476-483, 1980.

4. Ottenbacher K: The effect of a controlled program of vestibular stimulation on the incidence of seizures in children with severe developmental delay. *Phys Occup Ther Pediatr* 2(2/3):25-34, 1982.

5. Ottenbacher K: Vestibular processing dysfunction in children with severe emotional and behavior disorders: A review. *Phys Occup Ther Pediatr* 2(1):3-12, 1982.

6. Ottenbacher K: Developmental implications of clinically applied vestibular stimulation: A review. *Phys Ther* 63:338-342, 1983.

7. Ottenbacher K, Petersen P: A meta analysis of applied vestibular stimulation research. *Phys Occup Ther Pediatr* 5(2/3):119-130, 1985.

Because of the posed link between vestibular dysfunction and motor delays, recent investigations have been exploring the effects of vestibular stimulation on the subsequent emergence of motor skills and postural adjustment responses. The results of these investigations revealed that programs of vestibular stimulation enhanced motor and postural development in normal neonates,[13-15] in premature infants,[16-18] in children with Down's syndrome and in normal controls,[19] and in children with cerebral palsy.[20] Sellick and Over,[21] however, recently reported that a program of vestibular stimulation with cerebral palsied children did not reveal statistically significant developmental gains beyond those observed in a control group. The findings of Sellick and Over[21] indicate the need for continued empirical investigation to establish the efficacy of vestibular stimulation procedures with developmentally disabled children.

Although the use of therapeutically applied vestibular and proprioceptive stimulation is becoming increasingly popular in clinic programs, the methods and parameters of such stimulation have not yet been delineated. The studies by Kantner and others[19] and Chee and others,[20] while demonstrating significant improvement in the motor and reflex function of developmentally delayed subjects receiving vestibular stimulation, used stimulation procedures which are generally not feasible in clinic settings. For example, those studies required a ratio of two adults for one child, the precise positioning of the child's head to isolate specific semicircular canals, and a darkened room which contained a specially adapted rotating chair. The majority of clinic settings do not possess the staff, space, equipment, or time to replicate these procedures. It is necessary, therefore, to determine if experimental procedures for producing effective vestibular stimulation can be sufficiently altered and accommodated to clinical settings. For the present study, it was decided to explore in a clinical setting the effects of delivering a less procedurally rigorous program of vestibular stimulation on the emergence of motor skills and postural reflexes in developmentally delayed children.

METHOD

Selection of Children

Subjects consisted of 38 severely developmentally delayed residents of the Arkansas Children's Colony, Conway Unit. The children, who ranged in age from 39 to 129 months, were all nonambulatory and functioning within the severe to profound range of mental retardation, as measured by state licensed psychologists. Fourteen of the children had a medical diagnosis of spastic cerebral palsy, six had a medical diagnosis of athetosis, eight evidenced hypotonicity, and ten were diagnosed as mixed or other.

Evaluations

All children were evaluated before and after therapy using the Peabody Developmental Motor Scales[22] and a reflex assessment adapted from Kreutzberg[23] and used in previous studies of vestibular stimulation.[15,20] The reflex test measures, on a 4-point ordinal scale, 17 reflexes and reactions which fall into four general categories: primitive, righting, protective, and equilibrium. The Peabody Developmental Motor Scale (PDMS) measures gross and fine motor performance in children 0 to 6 years of age. This instrument was selected because it incorporates the assessment of a fine gradation of performance, ranging from total dependence to complete independence. These gradations enable the quantification of progress within each developmental age and facilitate the assessment of neuromotor performance in children whose severe motor impairments prevent them from making large gains in terms of moving from one developmental level or age to the next.

In addition, all children were assessed for the presence of spasticity. This assessment was made during the reflex testing and was confirmed by checking information contained in each subject's medical chart. The criteria used to determine spasticity was hyperactive stretch and deep tendon reflexes and the presence of exaggerated muscle tonus. All children determined to exhibit spasticity on initial testing also had medical diagnoses of spastic muscle tonus in their medical records.

Procedure and Apparatus

Following the initial evaluations, all children were paired as closely as possible on the variables of motor and reflex scores, age, sex, and type of muscle tonus present. One member of each pair was then randomly assigned to a treatment or control group. The treatment group received a program of vestibular stimulation followed by sensorimotor therapy from the PDMS program three times per week for about 40 minutes per period. The control subjects were taken to the treatment room and spent the entire therapy time of approximately 40 minutes receiving the PDMS program of sensorimotor activities. The PDMS sensorimotor program[22] focuses on the teaching of specific gross and fine motor skills which are geared to each child's level of motor development, as determined from pretest PDMS scores. The PDMS sensorimotor activities for the treatment group lasted approximately 10-15 minutes and followed a 25-30 minute program of vestibular stimulation. Each vestibular treatment session was administered with the child in two different positions. Initially, the child was positioned upright in a suspended car seat (Figure 1) and rotated first in a clockwise and then in a counterclockwise direction. Then the child was positioned supine in a suspended net hammock (Figure 2) and rotated the same as when seated. Rotation was done manually at approximately 100°/sec., or 17 revolutions per minute, for one minute (as adapted from the research of Clark and others[15] and Chee and others[20]). Rotation was timed by a stopwatch. This procedure was repeated, resulting in a total of two clockwise and two counterclockwise rotations while seated and then while supine. A rest period of at least one minute separated all rotations. The remainder of the time allotted for vestibular stimulation (25-30 minutes) was used in positioning and securing the subject in the apparatus. Children were monitored closely to observe any rapid changes in respiration rate, heart rate, or skin color. The rate of rotation employed

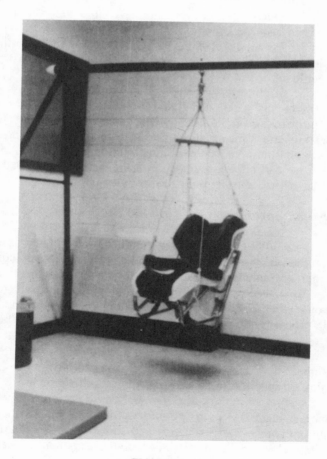

FIGURE 1

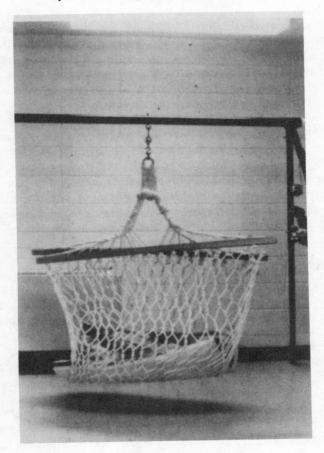

FIGURE 2

was relatively slow, and the majority of the subjects appeared to enjoy the stimulation and to be relaxed by it. Precautions were followed as outlined by Clark and Shuer.[24]

Initially, an attempt was made to regulate each child's head position while he/she was in the treatment apparatus in order to isolate and stimulate more specifically the semicircular canals; however, after starting the vestibular stimulation, it became obvious that strict head positioning would require more elaborate equipment than was available in most clinics. Therefore, no further attempts were made to control head position precisely.

Treatment and control groups received equivalent amounts of time in therapy, approximately 100-120 minutes per week per child. Therapy was continued for a period of 13 weeks, at which time the PDMS and reflex assessment was readministered. All treatment was carried out by two therapists and two aides who had been instructed in the therapeutic procedures. Evaluations were conducted by a state-licensed therapist experienced in pediatric assessment who was uninvolved in the initial assignment of subjects to conditions. No reliability estimates were available for either the PDMS or the reflex assessment.

RESULTS

Four children, two from the treatment condition and two controls, were dropped from the study. One child contracted an ear infection, which appeared to be aggravated by the vestibular stimulation; two children were released from the residential facility; and the fourth child required hospitalization for a respiratory infection. Data for the remaining 34 children (17 treatment and 17 control) were utilized for analysis.

The matching procedure resulted in groups of approximately equal developmental ability. Pretesting revealed mean gross motor developmental ages of 7.23 months and 7.41 months for the control and treatment groups, respectively. The mean developmental age for fine motor ability was 7.59 months for the control group and 7.94 months for the treatment group.

Motor development scores were calculated for both pretherapy and posttherapy performance in gross and fine motor tasks. These scores were computed by adding criteria scores for each item from the subject's basal to ceiling scores on the PDMS. These scores could be converted into developmental age equivalents (see Folio and DuBose[22]). In addition, for each subject a reflex test score was computed by adding the points scored on each of the 17 reflex measures. Gain scores for each child were then determined for the fine motor, gross motor, and reflex measures. Figure 3 compares graphically the mean gain scores for the two groups on the three dependent variables. The gain scores, which were computed by subtracting pretest scores from posttest scores, were statistically compared to see if differences in neuromotor performance existed between the control and treatment conditions. Because the data were based on ordinal scales, a nonparametric statistical technique, the Mann-Whitney U, was utilized for data analysis. The results of these analyses are reported in Table 1 and reveal that significant differences in neuromotor performance were noted for all three dependent variables. For gross motor, fine motor, and reflex integration measures, the treatment group made increases in *gain* scores that were significantly greater than those made by the control group.

In addition, rank order and point-biserial correlations were computed for all subjects between the three dependent variables using the gain

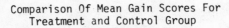

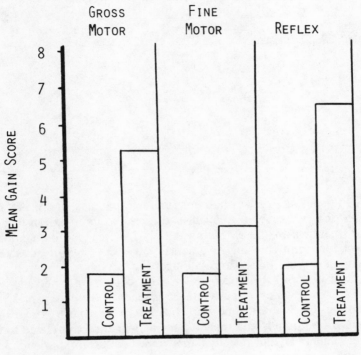

FIG. 3

scores and the extraneous variables of age, sex, and presence or absence of spasticity taken at the beginning of the study. This analysis revealed significant correlations between gross motor and age (rho $-.38\ p < .01$), gross motor and fine motor (rho $.33\ p < .05$), reflex and gross motor (rho $.60 < .001$), gross motor and spasticity ($r_{pb}\ .39\ p < .01$), and reflex and spasticity ($r_{pb}\ .32\ p < .05$). None of the other correlations was statistically significant.

DISCUSSION AND CONCLUSION

The treatment and habilitation of severely handicapped children is a complex problem facing health professionals, educators, and parents. In the past, severely multiply handicapped children were often confined to institutions, where there was limited opportunity for therapeutic intervention. Recently, however, with the emphasis on the rights of all handi-

Table I

Means and Significance Levels For Dependent Variables

Dependent Variable	Mean Gain Scores		U-Value	
	Treatment Group	Control Group		
Fine Motor	3.06	1.71	93	p < .05+
	2.33 SD	1.93 SD		
Gross Motor	5.24	1.71	62.5	p < .01+
	3.70 SD	2.14 SD		
Reflex	6.53	2.00	52	p < .001+
	4.50 SD	1.97 SD		
+ One tailed				

capped persons to realize their maximum capacities, there has been a growing drive to develop relevant and effective intervention techniques for the treatment of the severely multiply handicapped population. The prospect for significant improvement for this population, however, has not been optimistic. For example, Piaget[25] reasoned that children who are affected in their sensorimotor period with both mental and motor handicaps are in double jeopardy of experiencing developmental delays. Confirming this is the recent work by Brassell,[26] who reported that the severity of both motor and mental handicaps is directly related to delays in development. That physically handicapped children experience sensory deprivation has been explained by Prescott,[27] who claims that these children are prevented from experiencing somatosensory (tactile, vestibular, and proprioceptive) stimulation because of reduced ability to interact with the environment. Related to this is the development of various forms of sensory stimulation in many currently popular therapies that attempt to ameliorate sensorimotor deficits in developmentally delayed children.[28]

The present study provided additional support for the use of sensory, particularly vestibular, stimulation in the treatment of developmental disabilities. In this study vestibular stimulation, applied in a controlled manner in a clinic setting, resulted in improved performance in gross and fine motor skills as well as facilitated reflex integration in severely developmentally delayed, multiply handicapped children. The largest gains found were in reflex integration, whereas the smallest gains were found in fine motor development. These findings are in agreement with the normal sequence of neuromotor development as outlined by Twitchell[3] and Peiper,[1] who postulate that various reflexes form the substrate underlying posture and coordinated voluntary movement and that changes within the reflex structure must precede development in the areas of gross motor and fine motor function. In addition, the correlational evidence which was computed across the treatment and control groups suggests that improvements obtained in motor function, particularly gross motor function, were closely related to reflex performance. Neuromotor gains in the area of gross motor skills appeared to be related to at least two external factors: age and the presence or absence of spasticity. Generally, the younger subjects achieved the greater gains in terms of neuromotor development, while those children without signs of spasticity appeared to make relatively better gross motor and reflex gains than those subjects with spasticity. In spite of the developmental changes made, as measured by increases in gain scores for the three dependent variables (gross and fine motor function, and reflex integration), there was only moderate progress made in terms of subjects' moving from one developmental age to the next in these same areas. Only three children in the treatment group improved sufficiently to move to a higher developmental age in any one of the three areas measured. Considering the severity of the disabilities in the population under investigation, however, it would be unrealistic to expect large shifts in developmental ages over such a relatively short period of study (13 weeks).

The difficulties in conducting research with a severely developmentally disabled population impose some restrictions regarding the interpretation of these results. The lack of standardized measuring instruments and the fact that reliability coefficients were not available for the measuring devices used introduce a certain amount of subjectivity and possible experimenter bias, limiting the implications of this study. A further limitation is the absence of a third control group that did not receive either sensorimotor or vestibular therapy. It is recognized that a certain amount of vestibular stimulation occurs naturally during handling in sensorimotor therapy. Ethical constraints, however, prevented the withholding of therapy from any subject; therefore, the relationship of vestibular or sensorimotor programs relative to no treatment intervention was unexplored. In addition, the small number of subjects and the variability of severe neuromotor disorders circumscribe the generalizability of these results. It is obvious that continued research is necessary to delineate the neuromotor effects of vestibular stimulation, to develop and explore the parameters of administration, and to identify further the clinical population most likely to benefit from a program of intervention employing vestibular stimulation.

REFERENCES

1. Peiper A: *Cerebral Function in Infancy and Early Childhood.* New York, Consultants Bureau, 1963.

2. Prechtl HFR, Beintema D. The neurological examination of the full term newborn infant. *Little Club Clinics in Developmental Medicine,* No. 12, London, Spastics Society, 1964.

3. Twitchell TE: Attitudinal reflexes. *Journal of the American Physical Therapy Association* 45:411-418, 1965.

4. Milani-Comparetti A, Gidoni EA: Pattern analysis of motor development and its disorders. *Developmental Medicine and Child Neurology* 9:625-630, 1967.

5. Rushworth G: On postural and righting reflexes. *Developmental Medicine and Child Neurology* 3:535-554, 1961.

6. Bobath B, Bobath K: *Motor Development in the Different Types of Cerebral Palsy.* London, W. Heinemann Books, 1975.

7. Sherrington CS: *The Integrative Action of the Nervous System.* New York, Charles Scribner and Sons, 1914.

8. Magnus R: Physiology of posture. *Lancet* 2:531-536, 585-588, 1926.

9. Roberts TDM: *Neurophysiology of Postural Mechanisms.* London, Butterworths, 1967.

10. Wilson VJ: The labyrinth, the brain and posture. *American Scientist* 63:325-332, 1975.

11. Torok N, Perlstein MA: Vestibular findings in cerebral palsy. *Annals of Otology, Rhinology and Laryngology* 71:51-67, 1962.

12. Molnar G: Analysis of motor disorder in retarded infants and young children. *American Journal of Mental Deficiency* 83:213-222, 1979.

13. Korner A, Thoman E: Visual alertness in neonates as evoked by maternal care. *Journal of Experimental Child Psychology* 10:67-78, 1972.

14. Gregg, CL, Haffner ME, Korner AF: The relative efficacy of vestibular proprioceptive stimulation and the upright position in enhancing the visual pursuits in neonates. *Child Development* 47:309-314, 1976.

15. Clark D, Kreutzberg J, Chee F: Vestibular stimulation influence on motor development in infants. *Science* 196:1228-1229, 1977.

16. Freedman D, Boverman H: The effects of kinesthetic stimulation and certain aspects of development in premature infants. *American Journal of Orthopsychiatry* 36:223-225, 1966.

17. Neal M: Vestibular stimulation and developmental behavior of the small premature infant. *Nursing Research Report* 3:3-5, 1968.

18. Solkoff N, Yaffe E, Weintraub D: Effects of handling on the subsequent development of premature infants. *Developmental Psychology* 1:765-768, 1969.

19. Kantner RM, Clark D, Allen LC, Chase M: Effects of vestibular stimulation on nystagmus response and motor performance in the developmentally delayed infant. *Physical Therapy* 56: 414-421, 1976.

20. Chee F, Kreutzberg J, Clark D: Semicircular canal stimulation in cerebral palsied children. *Physical Therapy* 58:1071-1075, 1978.

21. Sellick KJ, Over R: Effects of vestibular stimulation on motor development of cerebral palsied children. *Developmental Medicine and Child Neurology* 22:476-483, 1980.

22. Folio R, DuBose RF: *Peabody Developmental Motor Scales.* Nashville, TN, George Peabody College for Teachers, 1974.

23. Kreutzberg J: *Effects of vestibular stimulation on the reflex and motor development in normal infants.* Ann Arbor, MI, *Dissertation Abstracts International,* 1976.

24. Clark FA, Shuer J: A clarification of sensory integrative therapy and its application to programming with retarded people. *Mental Retardation* 16:227-232, 1978.

25. Piaget J: *The Origins of Intelligence in Children.* New York, International University Press, 1952.

26. Brassell WR: Intervention with handicapped infants: Correlates of progress. *Mental Retardation* 16:18-22, 1978.

27. Prescott JW: Somatosensory deprivation and its relationship to the blind, in Jastrzembska Z (ed): *The Effects of Blindness and Other Impairments on Early Development.* New York, The American Foundation for the Blind, 1976.

28. Pearson PH, Williams CE (eds): *Physical Therapy Services in the Developmental Disabilities.* Springfield, IL, C. C. Thomas, 1972.

PART 6:
RESOURCES FOR RESEARCH

No one person has all of the skills to be an excellent clinician, researcher, statistician, writer, politician, and whatever additional roles are necessary to see a research project from conceptualization to publication. Collaboration takes care of that problem because it enables people with varying skills and abilities to come together, to share their skills, to give and receive encouragement, and to achieve goals that none of the individuals could achieve alone. Collaborations do not need to be permanent and, instead of fostering dependency, they can provide a basis for learning which can lead to acquisition of independent research abilities for all of the members.

Many ways are available to start a research collaboration. Sometimes it can develop from mutual interest in testing a new intervention or from a special interest group that meets to discuss common needs and goals. For therapists who work alone, a number of individuals and resources may be consulted. Individuals who work in communities with a college might want to collaborate with other professionals who have already developed research competencies. Many academic professionals (such as other allied health professionals, special educators, psychologists, or physicians) are looking for accessible clinical subject pools. Bargains can be struck with these individuals to allow access to subject populations, providing assistance is given with the design and data analysis of your own study. Many psychology, occupational therapy, nursing, or special education departments need locations for training students in such areas as behavioral analysis or clinical observation. Again, bargains can be struck whereby students can be used to gather data for you while they simultaneously develop clinical skills. Or, you can agree to the placement of college students in your clinic, providing you can have access to the college computer and statistical consultation.

Similarly, many studies can be couched within other studies so that collaborators might use the same subject pool while gathering twice the amount of data. (Be careful that such a procedure is reported, as the added assessments could affect the results of a study.) Such an arrangement is often possible with graduate students who may be willing to perform some volunteer work in order to gain access to subject pools. Collaboration can be fun, can sustain efforts when individual efforts flag, and can enhance problem-solving in a more innovative, versatile manner than can one person alone. Certainly collaborations work best when the agendas of all the participants are explicit and negotiated. (The politics of collaboration are discussed in more detail in Part 3.)

REPORTING RESULTS OF A RESEARCH PROJECT

Reporting the results of an investigation is not a privilege but an obligation. Many specialists may benefit from the findings of your investigation. The nature of many clinical fields is that commonly a single therapist comprises a department. These individuals are isolated and need the input of other colleagues. Any findings by other professionals in their field may be significant to these clinicians who need in-service programs, regional conferences and local meetings for support, stimulation and encouragement.

Reporting your findings can be done in many ways, informally among colleagues at in-service programs, national or regional conferences, or in published form. Similarly, the many outlets for publication range from professional journals to special interest section newsletters.

HOW TO PUBLISH A RESEARCH ARTICLE

One of the best guarantees of publishing research is to use an adequate, well-developed research design and procedure. One of the most unfortunate circumstances encountered by the enthusiastic novice researcher is that he or she collects enormous amounts of data and then doesn't know what to do with it. Good research is developed ahead of time: potential problems are anticipated and solutions are considered; the nature of the data to be collected is understood, and the statistics are determined; potential results are considered along with their "fit" with accompanying theory or already published research in the same area; potential confounds, conflicting interpretations, and alternative explanations are considered, and *then* the study can begin. A good study is completely formulated, with an introduction and consideration of findings, so that the final steps involve gathering and analyzing the data, and discussing the implications of the results.

One of the ways to simplify the decisions required for developing a design, procedure, and data analysis is to conduct research in an area where that has already been done. Replicating research is important. It is valuable to conduct a study similar to one that has already been conducted except for manipulating one characteristic of the independent *or* dependent variables, *or* a characteristic of the subject population. (The independent variable in an experiment is typically the intervention, whereas the dependent variable is the measure of change.) Thus, a previously published study can essentially be replicated, except for altering the intensity or frequency of the intervention, *or* using a different measurement or assessment tool. These are examples for experimental designs but as many other examples for obtaining normative data using other procedures could be cited.

For discussions about the types of research, and for more information about research in a specific field, the student is referred to other resources regarding research, experimental design, and statistics. Some references are included at the end of this section.

Finally, once a study has been conducted, a location for publication must be found. If the researcher is experienced, often the study is already written with an audience in mind. If the study is not yet written, a little extra research must be done. First, consider the audience you want to address. Is it a specialized group of therapists or educators, e.g., only those who work in mental health, pediatrics, linguistics, or in parent counseling? If so, you might want to orient your study for a journal most likely to reach other similar specialists. If your study is of general interest, you may want to submit it to a journal with a wider orientation such as: *Journal of Learning Disabilities, Perceptual-Motor Skills*, or *Child Development*. If your study is preliminary or based on only a few subjects, it might be more appropriate as "Research in Progress", or a "Clinical Concern" in a specialized journal such as *Physical and Occupational Therapy in Pediatrics* or as a "Brief Report" in *Occupational Therapy Journal of Research*. Special interest newsletters also publish clinically relevant articles that may not be subjected to the close scrutiny or editorial review of a journal article. The ultimate decision regarding where to send a manuscript will depend on the audience you want to address. One way to make a decision regarding where to publish is to determine if your bibliographic references were published in a common journal. If so, that journal would probably be interested in similar research. Another political decision is based on the projected readership or prestige of a particular journal. If you are a new therapist or academician who is trying to establish a reputation within a certain area, then you would be wise to publish in a journal where your name will be recognized by other professionals in your field.

Once a decision is made regarding where to submit the manuscript for consideration, the manuscript must be written in the style appropriate for the journal. Different journals have different editorial styles as well as approaches. Some journals have style manuals that can be obtained from editors or are available in bookstores. Sometimes editorial policies can be gleaned from information included on the flyleaf of the journal in addition to close inspection of other studies published in that journal. Editorial/author guides should be consulted, as a manuscript may be returned because of lack of conformity to a journal's style. Journals also have different philosophies or approaches which usually are stated on the editorial page. This also can be determined by looking at the types and content of articles that are published in the journal. Often it helps, before writing a final draft to submit for publication to a specific journal, to sit down and read several issues of the journal. The style and approach will then become evident to you, and you may find it easier to adopt that journal's particular "voice".

Probably the biggest piece of advice regarding getting a manuscript published is to be persistent. Research manuscripts are often rejected. When a manuscript is submitted to a journal, the editor typically sends it to a number of reviewers, who read, critique, and make recommendations regarding the style, content, and suitability of the manuscript for publication. The editor, based on feedback from the reviewers, will then notify you whether the submission is accepted, accepted providing revisions are made, or rejected. Like anything that depends on the input of a number of people, reviewed manuscripts always require some change. Sometimes the changes are minimal (but that is rare!). Most of the time, manuscripts have to be revised, data may need to be re-analyzed, or new theories and references need to be considered. Reviews are helpful, and they often round-out a narrowly focused study. Sometimes manuscripts are rejected, but the reviewers advice can be taken, papers can be re-submitted, re-reviewed and accepted. To get an article published requires patience and persistence. If one journal rejects your manuscript, try another journal. If that journal rejects it, consider the feedback, make revisions, and try another. If your study is important, you will find a forum for sharing it. This may necessitate re-writing, some frustration, and accepting criticism, but is often worth the effort. If you truly feel that your study has been misunderstood or improperly reviewed, contact the editor and seek his or her advice.

RESEARCH ASSISTANCE AND RESOURCES

Many national organizations offer research assistance to therapists. For example, the Foundation for Physical Therapy (FPT) and The American Occupational Therapy Foundation (AOTF) support the conduct of research in their professions and periodically offer grant support for a variety of individuals. Many organizations offer workshops pertaining to research, and both the APTA and the AOFT have regional research consultants who can offer advice on the development of research projects.

Other professionals offer advice in the form of articles or editorials, which are frequently published (or in the case of books, advertised) in newsletters or journals. Many of these provide excellent suggestions and information regarding various stages (and forms) of research. Some of these are listed below:

Office of Professional Research Services, American Occupational Therapy Foundation, 1383 Piccard Drive, Rockville, MD, 20850. (Telephone: 914-834-5760) Associate Executive Director for Research and Education (Eugene Michels), American Physical Therapy Association, 1111 N. Fairfax Street, Alexandria, VA, 22314. (Telephone: 703-684-2782)

JOURNALS

(Note: The following addresses are subject to change, and for the most recent contacts, specific journals should be consulted.)

Occupational Therapy in Health Care: A Journal of Contemporary Practice. Haworth Press. Editor: Florence S. Cromwell, OTR, OTHC, 1179 Yocum Street, Pasadena, CA 91103

Occupational Therapy in Mental Health. Haworth Press. Editor: Diane Gibson, OTR, Director, Activity Therapy Department, The Sheppard and Enoch Pratt Hospital, Towson, MD 21204

Physical and Occupational Therapy in Geriatrics. Haworth Press. Co-editors: Jean M. Kiernat, OTR, and Betty Risteen Hasselkus, OTR, Center for Health Sciences, Occupational Therapy Program, 1300 University Avenue, Madison, WI 53706

Physical and Occupational Therapy in Pediatrics. Haworth Press. Co-editors: Suzann K. Campbell, PhD and Irma J. Wilhelm, MS, Department of Medical Allied Health Professions, Medical School Wing E 222H, University of North Carolina at Chapel Hill, Chapel Hill, NC 27514

Physical Therapy. Editor: Marilyn Lister, American Physical Therapy Association, 1111 N. Fairfax Street, Alexandria, VA 22314

Physical Therapy in Health Care. Haworth Press. Co-editors: Mary C. Singleton, PhD, PT, Department of Medical Allied Health Professions, University of North Carolina at Chapel Hill, Medical School Wing E 222H, Chapel Hill, NC 27514 and Eleanor F. Branch, PhD, PT, Department of Physical Therapy, Box 3405, Duke University Medical Center, Durham, NC 27710

The American Journal of Occupational Therapy. Editor: Elaine Viseltear, 616 Tanner Marsh Road, Guilford, CT 06437

The Occupational Therapy Journal of Research. The American Occupational Therapy Association, Inc. Editor: Charles H. Christiansen, Occupational Therapy Program, 7703 Floyd Curl Drive, San Antonio, TX 78284; manuscripts to: Associate Editor: Cynthia Berchulc, Substation 1, Box 86, Galveston, TX 77550

Regarding additional journals, the following may be consulted: *Authors Guide to Journals in the Health Field*, or *Author's Guide to Journals in Nursing and Related Fields*, both available from: The Haworth Press, Inc., 28 East 22nd Street, New York, NY 10010

BOOKS

Barlow DH, Hayes SC, Nelsen RO: *The Scientist-Practitioner: Research and Accountability in Clinical and Educational Settings.* New York, Pergamon Press, 1984

Bruning JL, Kintz BL: *Computational Handbook of Statistics, 2nd ed.* Glenview, IL, Scott, Foresman & Co., 1977

Cox RC, West WL: *Fundamentals of Research for Health Professionals.* Laurel, MD, RAMSCO Publishing Co., 1982

Currier DP: *Elements of Research in Physical Therapy, 2nd ed.* Baltimore, Williams & Wilkins, 1984

Day RA: *How to Write and Publish a Scientific Paper, 2nd ed.* Philadelphia, ISI Press, 1983

Ethridge DA, McSweeney M: *Research in Occupational Therapy.* Dubuque, IA, Kendall/Hunt Publishing Co., 1971

Jantzen AC: *Research: The Practical Approach for Occupational Therapy.* Laurel, MD, RAMSCO Publishing Co., 1981

Glaser EM, Abelson HH, Garrison KN: *Putting Knowledge to Use: Facilitating the Diffusion of Knowledge and the Implementation of Planned Change.* San Francisco, Jossey-Bass Inc. Publishers, 1983

Mahoney MJ: *Scientist as Subject: The Psychological Imperative.* Cambridge, MA, Ballinger Publishing Co., 1976

Ottenbacher K: *Evaluating Clinical Change: Strategies for Occupational and Physical Therapists.* Baltimore, Williams & Wilkins, in press

Payton OD: *Research: The Validation of Clinical Practice.* Philadelphia, FA Davis, 1979

Publication Manual of the American Psychological Association, 3rd ed. Washington, DC, American Psychological Association, 1982

Richardson FR: *Author's Style Guide to The American Journal of Occupational Therapy*. Rockville, MD, American Occupational Therapy Association, 1979

Stein F: *Anatomy of Research in Allied Health, 2nd ed*. Cambridge, MA, Schenkman Publishing Co., 1980

Stylebook/Editorial Manual of the AMA. Littleton, MA, PSG Publishing Co., Inc., 1976

Style Manual: Physical Therapy, Journal of the American Physical Therapy Association, 4th ed. Washington, DC, American Physical Therapy Association, 1976

JOURNAL ARTICLES

Basmajian JV: Research or retrench: The rehabilitation professions challenged. *Phys Ther* 55:607-610, 1975

Carroll RS, Miller A, Ross B, et al.: Research as an impetus to improved treatment. *Arch Gen Psychol* 37:377-380, 1980

Christiansen CH: Editorial. Research: An economic imperative. *Occup Ther J Res* 3:195-198, 1983

Conine TA: Dilemmas of research in occupational therapy. *Am J Occup Ther* 26:81-84, 1972

Cox R: The case study method of research: Introduction. *Sensory Integration Specialty Section Newsletter* 4:1-4, 1981

Crocker LM: Linking research to practice: Suggestions for reading a research article. *Am J Occup Ther* 31:34-39, 1977

Dumholdt EA, Malone TR: Evaluating research literature: The educated clinician. *Phys Ther* 65:487-491, 1985

The Foundation: Research in occupational therapy. It's everybody's responsibility. *Am J Occup Ther* 33:666-667, 1979

Greenstein LE: Teaching research: An introduction to statistical concepts and research terminology. *Am J Occup Ther* 34:320-327, 1980

Hacker B: Single subject research: Strategies in occupational therapy. Parts I and II. *Am J Occup Ther* 34:103-108, 169-175, 1980

Hasselkus BR, Safrit MJ: Measurement in occupational therapy. *Am J Occup Ther* 30:429-436, 1976

Kielhofner G: Qualitative research: Part one. Paradigmatic grounds and issues of reliability and validity. *Occup Ther J Res* 2:67-70, 1982

Kielhofner G: Qualitative research: Part two: Methodological approaches and relevance to occupational therapy. *Occup Ther J Res* 2:150-164, 1982

Kispert CP: Reading Tips. Introduction to hypotheses testing. *Phys Ther* 65:1544-1550, 1985

Mann WC: Survey methods. *Am J Occup Ther* 39:640-648, 1985

Marks RG: Choosing the appropriate design and analysis of a research project. *Occup Ther Ment Health* 1:69-76, 1980

Morse JA: Critical analysis of research. *Sensory Integration Specialty Section Newsletter* 4:3-4, 1981

Ottenbacher K: Statistical power and research in occupational therapy. *Occup Ther J Res* 2:13-26, 1982

Ottenbacher K: The significance of power and the power of significance: Recommendations for occupational therapy research. *Occup Ther J Res* 4:38-50, 1984

Powell JN: Advice to novice researchers on preparing grant proposals for AOTF. *Am J Occup Ther* 37:203-204, 1983

Slater SB: The design of clinical research. *Phys Ther* 46:265-273, 1966

Stein F: Evaluating psychiatric treatment methods through clinical trials research. *Occup Ther Ment Health* 1:1-14, 1980

West WL: Research seminar. *Am J Occup Ther* 30:477-478, 1976

Witt, PL: Reading Tips. Comparing two sample means: t tests. *Phys Ther* 65:1731-1733, 1985

Witt PL: Research Writing Tips. *Phys Ther* 60:93-95, 209-210, 477-479, 805-806, 929-930, 1049-1050, 1980

Yerxa EJ, Gilfoyle E: The Foundation. Research seminar. *Am J Occup Ther* 30:509-511, 1976

Zimmerman JP: Statistical data and their use. *Phys Ther* 49:301-302, 1969

Many students, clinicians, or novice researchers feel that conducting and publishing research are idealistic and unattainable personal goals. Supporting this are the beliefs that research must be conducted independently and that every investigator must carve out his or her own specific and unique area of study. We hope that one of the functions of this anthology has been to dispel those beliefs.

Many of the studies in this anthology are the result of collaboration between individuals who each brought his or her own strengths and talents to the research tasks. Each of us learned from one another and benefitted from working together. The ideas generated by a group are, indeed, more creative and numerous than those produced by individuals working in isolation. Collaboration promotes growth, innovation, and the development of unique research approaches and solutions. As this anthology demonstrates, clinicians can simultaneously work independently and collaboratively toward seeking answers to the myriad questions generated by clinical research.

This anthology includes a series of studies which were designed to address systematically specific issues (e.g., vestibular and proprioceptive variables, ocular fixation, and behavioral problems) in a focussed area of study (clinical assessment of learning disabilities). Our intention has been to use these studies to illustrate how single investigations can spawn other relevant research. Unfortunately, many novice researchers feel that their research will be valid only if they design new test instruments to examine the effects of unique interventions on previously unexamined dependent variables. Such studies are particularly cumbersome, time-consuming, and, unfortunately, often inconclusive.

We have no intention of discouraging innovative research. There is a pressing need for clinical researchers to develop new, valid and reliable instruments specifically designed to assess the variables under study in their fields. New measuring instruments, however, take time to be developed, pilot tested, and validated. In addition, novel independent and dependent variables must be isolated, explored, and placed within a context of relevant literature. New therapies need to be thoroughly examined, and normative studies are needed to explore the diverse dependent variables generated with new assessment tools. Research is methical; and conclusions drawn from it are slow in coming. Answers are not obtained by single investigations, and the nature of experimentation is that studies designed to examine too many variables at once will result in many more questions than answers. As was illustrated in Part 5, informative studies often replicate a previously published methodology while varying one factor at a time, e.g., the type of clinical population, a characteristic of the independent variable, a related but different dependent variable. For example, Ottenbacher has suggested how different studies could be designed to explore the effectiveness of therapeutic vestibular stimulation. Such studies would systematically examine the parameters of stimulation, the effect of subjects' positioning during stimulation, and the effects of specific stimulation on various ages and diagnostic types of subjects.[1]

While we researchers tend to expect each new study to provide answers to multi-variable problems, the nature of research is that it results in more questions. A collection of systematically designed clinical studies addresses those questions, one at a time, with the goals of identifying specific parameters and isolating variables involved in effective intervention. A body of literature which has systematically examined specific variables enables clinicians to make more conclusive statements about treatment effectiveness than could be done with collections of single, isolated, unrelated studies. Sound research conclusions are based on a context that contains investigations and replications by numerous researchers with differing orientations.[2] Replications are not only easy to design; in science, they are necessary.

The narrative of this anthology, as well as the discussion sections of individual studies reprinted here, provides many suggestions for continued research in this field. We strongly encourage interested readers to develop spin-offs and replications of these studies. We hope that this anthology will encourage some of you either to begin collaborating with colleagues or to develop your own research investigations, and to provide us with additional insights about clinical assessment and intervention.

REFERENCES

1. Ottenbacher K: Developmental implications of clinically applied vestibular stimulation: A review. *Phys Ther* 63:338-342, 1983.

2. Ottenbacher K, Short MA: Message from the editors. *Phys Occup Ther Pediatr* 5(2/3):1-3, 1985.

Subject Index

A

abstract (of a study) 10
academic abilities, deficits 1,45,65,70,71,
    87,90,95,102,105,109,111-113,124
acknowledgements (in research) 60,63
activities 5,6,57,73,94,95,100
adult tests 54,94
age (as variable in assessment) 31,69,78,80,
    85,114,115,122,128,136,139,150
aggression 79,80
allied health 11
American Journal of Occupational Therapy
    (AJOT) 13-19
American Occupational Therapy Foundation
    (AOTF) 14,16,144,145
American Physical Therapy Assn. 145
applied research 27
Arkansas Children's Colony 132
arousal 22,55,80,101,120,124
asymmetrical tonic neck reflex (ATNR)
    35-46
authorship in research 59-60
autism 74,124

B

balance 1,22,58,87,101,119,121,131
    assessment 50
    dynamic 24-55
    standing 24-55,119,121
Barany's test 54,113
baseline 61,62,95
behavioral problems (& l.d.) 1,57,58,65,
    73-81,90,124
bibliography 143
body image (see self image)

C

caloric stimulation, tests 28,54
case studies 15
celeration line 99-101
cerebellum 66,111
cerebral palsy 131,132
chi-square 16,17,30
clinical measures, observation, assessment
    1,2,5,6,29-55,57,59,71,87,96,105,
    119-125,149

co-contraction 30-46,96,101
collaborative research 2,3,17,57,59,60,141,
    149
control (in research 17,59,61-63,94,102,
    127,138,139
correlational research 9,15,21,22,45,49,57,
    69,71,108,109,112,128,136

D

data collection 59,62
descriptive research 9,15
development 74,112,131
developmental delays 28,131
Devereau Elementary School Behavior
    Rating Scale 74
draw-a-person test 5,83
dyslexia 35,66,74,112,124

E

East Tennessee Children's Rehabilitation
    Center 3,4,57
editorial policies 143,144
education (see academics)
efficacy of treatment 4,14,25,54,57,61,66,
    71,86,87,94,102,107,127,139,143,150
electronystamography 94,113
emotional problems & l.d.
    (see behavior problems)
equilibrium (see balance)
ethics of research 3,58,60,63,107,127,139
experimental research, method 9,15,84,85,
    94,127-139,143
eye-hand coordination (see perceptual motor)

F

fine motor 131
fixation (see ocular, visual)
Floor Ataxia Test Battery 50,52
Foundation for Physical Therapy 144

G

graphs (presenting data) 95,100,102
gross motor 131,136

Index of Names